stuttering therapy: transfer and maintenance

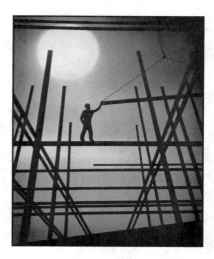

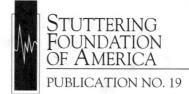

STUTTERING
FOUNDATION
OF AMERICA

PUBLICATION NO. 19

First Printing—1982
Second Printing—1988
Third Printing—1990
Fourth Printing—1994
Fifth Printing—1996

Published by

Stuttering Foundation of America
P.O. Box 11749
Memphis, Tennessee 38111-0749

ISBN 0-933388-19-5

To the Clinician

The real challenge for every clinician working with stutterers is to carry out therapy in such a way that the progress made in the clinical situation, be it that of increased fluency or of modified attitudes, is transferred to real life situations and maintained over time.

Because of the crucial role that transfer and maintenance play in stuttering therapy, the Stuttering Foundation of America held a week-long conference of leading authorities in order to discuss this important subject in depth. The principles and procedures described here are the result of this conference.

We believe your clinical effectiveness will be enhanced by careful consideration of the goals and processes described by these authors.

Jane Fraser
President

Stuttering Foundation of America

Conference Participants

Einer Boberg, Ph.D.

    Professor, Department of Speech Pathology and Audiology, University of Alberta, Edmondton. Editorial Board, *Journal of Fluency Disorders.* Editorial Consultant, *Journal of Speech and Hearing Disorders.*

Edward G. Conture, Ph.D.

    Associate Professor, Audiology and Speech Pathology, Syracuse University. Associate Editor, *Journal of Speech and Hearing Research.* Editorial Consultant, *Journal of Speech and Hearing Disorders.*

Malcolm Fraser

    Director, Stuttering Foundation of America.

Hugo H. Gregory, Ph.D., Conference Chairman

    Professor and Head, Speech and Language Pathology, Department of Communicative Disorders, Northwestern University. Editorial Board, *Journal of Fluency Disorders.* Editorial Consultant, *Journal of Speech and Hearing Disorders.*

Jane Fraser, Editor

    President, Stuttering Foundation of America.

Conference Participants

William H. Perkins, Ph.D.

> Professor, Communication Arts and Science, Director, Intensive Therapy Program for Stuttering, University of Southern California. Editorial Consultant, *Journal of Speech and Hearing Disorders.*

Joseph G. Sheehan, Ph.D.

> Professor of Psychology, Director, Psychology Speech Clinic, University of California, Los Angeles (UCLA). Editorial Consultant, *Journal of Speech and Hearing Disorders, Journal of Communication Disorders.*

Elisabeth Versteegh-Vermeij

> Logopedist, Stichting Stottertherapie Doetinchemse Methode, Utrecht, The Netherlands.

Dean E. Williams, Ph.D.

> Professor, Speech Pathology and Audiology, University of Iowa. Editorial Board, *Journal of Communication Disorders.* Editorial Consultant, *Journal of Speech and Hearing Disorders.*

Contents

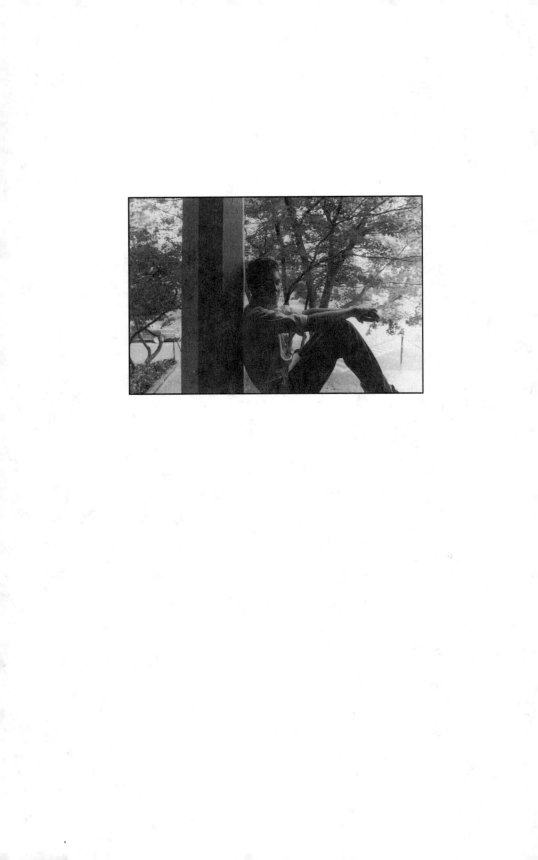

Preface

Hal is a 26 year old stutterer participating in a four-week intensive therapy program. Lois, age 13, receives therapy at junior high school. Nine year old Joe is enrolled with the school clinician for two 50 minute sessions each week. Bill, age four, considered a beginning stutterer, is seen along with his parents at the local college speech clinic.

With each of these cases, regardless of their age, the modification of stuttering and the production of increased fluency may not be particularly difficult. The challenge lies in carrying out therapy in such a way that modified speech is generalized or transferred to real life situations and then maintained over time.

During the last fifteen years, clinicians and researchers have given increased attention to defining the issues involved in effective transfer and maintenance of change. Presently, clinicians working with persons such as Hal, Lois, Joe, and Bill recognize more clearly the inadequacy of therapy that does not focus from the very beginning upon the goals of facilitating change outside the clinical situation, dealing with regression, and continuing the process of change. In work with children, the parents and other significant adults must be helped in order to maintain and extend modifications of their own behavior.

The contributors to this book discuss the principles and procedures that are crucial, in their view, to transfer and maintenance, or related directly to the process. They have some differences in beliefs about the nature of stuttering and have, therefore, had somewhat different experiences in therapy. We accept this. Our objective is to enhance the practicing clinician's realistic understanding of stuttering and stuttering therapy. Of course, clinicians have to filter what they read here through their own experience.

Definitions

Transfer of behavior change involves the occurrence or acquisition of changes in behavior in situations other than where the previous learning took place. In stuttering therapy, this most frequently refers to communicative responses being made in the natural, real-life environment following changes in the clinical situation. Thus, we speak of transfer from one situation to another. Responses transferred may be overt behavioral, including speech, and more covert attitudinal ones. Stimulus generalization enhances transfer, but clinicians also plan activities in which responses made successfully in one situation are practiced in another.

Maintenance of behavior change refers to the continuation or persistence of speech and attitudinal changes over time. It is the opposite of regression or relapse. Maintenance is related to the effectiveness of therapy in general, but clinicians also plan specific activities aimed toward the retention of therapeutic effects. Continuing the process of transfer is probably important in maintenance and maintaining gains enhances transfer.

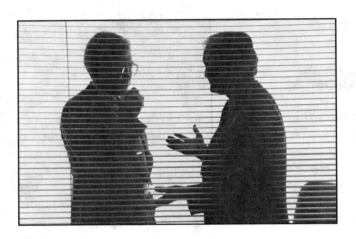

chapter one

The General Problem of Change

by Edward G. Conture, Ph.D.

Not everybody cares about that which we want them to learn. A cliché, perhaps, a platitude, maybe, but true nonetheless. Their unwillingness to learn not only involves formal learning situations like school, but also follows them out into the "real world." Such unwillingness even influences their ability to learn about themselves. These individuals, be they stutterers or non-stutterers, may complain that they don't like this or that aspect of themselves but when it comes down to actually changing these aspects, they "refuse to change."

In a popular book, Buscaglia discusses three issues involved with changing one's self or one's behavior. First, the individual must be dissatisfied with him or herself. Second, the person must make a decision to change that which is dissatisfying. Third, and most important we think in terms of transfer, the person must make a conscious dedication to the ". . . process of growth and change." It would seem that many stutterers, in and out of therapy, fulfill at least the first requirement for change: they are dissatisfied with their speech and themselves. A smaller group, those who probably come to our diagnostics, have met the second requirement: they have decided to change their speech. However, the smallest group yet, those for whom transfer, while not easy, is far less than insurmountable, have consciously committed themselves to the actions and behaviors necessary to change themselves and their behaviors.

We make the assumption that stutterers' ability to learn and transfer that learning is influenced by the same factors that influence non-stutterers. This assumption helps us gain perspective on why some stutterers are able to establish and transfer change while some who actually establish change seem unable to transfer it. Specifically, it seems quite probably that certain issues — (1) effort, (2) familiarity and (3) memory — influence everyone's learning and transfer of learning, stutterers and normally fluent speakers alike. We might describe the impact these issues have on learning and transfer by saying, "It's hard to remember to do something new." In other words, the problem of transfer and maintenance of change in stuttering therapy is most appropriately viewed within the broader context of human learning and then maintaining that learning.

Below we will describe some of these general issues which we believe impact learning and transfer of learning. Following that, we will discuss some "personality characteristics," and specific adjustment or coping mechanisms which can also influence the way a stutterer will decide and then commit himself to change of speech and self. These discussions will lead into specific discussion of transfer and how we think it may be best enhanced. First let us return to the three general issues (effort, familiarity and memory) that would seem capable of influencing human learning and transfer of that learning.

Transfer: Problems in General
Effort

When we consider the basics of whether a stutterer is or is not going to change his or her speech outside the clinic we are getting down to the fundamental question "Is it worth it?" This question probably means to the stutterer something like "Is more fluent speech worth the work, effort, and sweat I must go through to produce it?" In a sense, the stutterer in therapy is like the athlete learning a sport. The athlete who "plays with desire," who wants to play well, who wants to win, is willing to put in the time, effort and thought necessary to learn the sport and sharpen his skills. The various costs such as never-ending practices, injuries, set-backs, and coach's criticism are worth it to such an athlete.

Unfortunately, for some of our clients who stutter, the costs of increased fluency are not worth the price. Some will simply not endure outside the clinic, on their own, the necessary vigilance, practice and frustration of trying to establish more fluent speech and more fluency-facilitating attitudes. Just today we heard a young adult stutterer say, ". . . I didn't realize I'd have to concentrate so much, its really hard . . . I'm not sure I can do it or find the time to do it." For these people, the "old" way, no matter how socially unacceptable, is easier and less effortful than the "new" way.

Familiarity

It is said that familiarity breeds contempt. This may be true in terms of personal relationships but we do not believe it to be true in terms of our own behavior. Perhaps we complain loudly about how much weight we have put on or how we must be more accepting of others but we daily continue to put on weight or negatively evaluate other people. Why? For one thing we are used to such actions on our part; we are familiar with ourselves and we don't, in the final analysis, really want to change.

Our familiarity with our own behavior makes us unconscious of it. Our behavior is a bit like the clothes we wear, once they are on we forget about them unless someone specifically calls our attention to them. It is human to be content with that which we know best regardless of our "uplifting" notions to the contrary. To truly change a behavior and use another in its stead is not an activity that one undertakes lightly. It takes courage, persistence and willingness to fail because we are most comfortable with the familiar, including our "unwanted" behaviors. How much easier to "forget" the unfamiliar and "remember" the familiar.

Memory

In many ways our professional and personal lives are spent trying to remember one thing or another — prepare for classes, pay bills on time (at least sometimes!), write clinical reports on time, relate a present client to a similar case from the past, be tolerant of those under personal stress, and so forth. We remember that which is of greatest short as well as long-run importance to us. However, give us half a chance and we'll forget everything we can that "clutters" our mind with what we feel is ancillary, useless, or superfluous.

To remember to do something, like ". . . speak much slower when I talk to Johnny during our dinner-time conversations," requires the doer to believe it relevant, capable of being done and of importance. Above all, the act of remembering, particularly something that is new or unfamiliar, requires effort. If it were easy we'd see a lot more of it going around than we do. What complicates our ability to remember things are some of the ways we've learned to adjust to, cope or deal with problems.

In a very interesting book, Vaillant discusses the fact that all individuals, no matter their personal or professional successes, have problems. Vaillant quotes Barron as saying that "Soundness is a way of reacting to problems, not an absence of them." What differs among people, according to Vaillant and Barron, is not the frequency and nature of their problems but the way in which they adjust, cope or react to these problems. As the following discussion will show, this issue — reaction to problems — is quite germane to the topic of transfer with stutterers.

Transfer: Problems with Adjustment Strategies

Stutterers will have problems with communication during as well as after therapy. To tell them otherwise is to engage in prevarication. When therapy is terminated, they will face difficult speaking situations and less than attentive listeners. They will not always be able to be as fluent, articulate, and "scintillating" as they might like. The stutterers' need to verbally express thoughts during less than optimal speaking situations will persist. What can and should change, if stutterers are to make a meaningful transfer of behavior to situations outside the clinic is the way they habitually react to these situations. We need to be very observant in our clinical appraisal of stutterers and the "methods" by which they react to their problems with speech, themselves and their environment. We must be particularly concerned, I believe, in terms of transfer, when we observe stutterers who **frequently** and **persistently** cope with, react or adjust to their speech and related problems with what has been described as (Vaillant):

16

(1) repression, (2) intellectualization, (3) projection or (4) reaction formation.

The first problematic means of reacting to problems is the adjustment mechanism Vaillant terms "repression." We've all experienced the client who "forgets" to practice or change his speech behaviors, particularly changing those inappropriate attitudes, beliefs of emotions which contribute to their speech concerns. One client, we'll call him Steve, could make all sorts of changes in the clinic, but each time he'd report back for therapy he seemed to "forget" everything he'd learned the previous session.

We'd patiently resume therapy, trying to help him modify his behaviors and beliefs, explaining how these two interacted, what they looked, sounded and felt like and encouraged him to practice changing them. No matter what we did in therapy, Steve never transferred his changed behavior. He seemed to have a continual "memory lapse" regarding what we did in therapy. He was, of course, still able to remember to respond to the outside environment with his "old" emotions but — and this is crucial — he was seemingly unable to remember the **ideas** in therapy that would allow him to change these responses. He just didn't seem capable of sensing the physiological tensions and behaviors necessary to change these events when outside the clinic. While it is never easy to do something new, Steve made it even harder by repressing most of our therapy ideas and procedures while at the same time retaining the emotional responses to the world that contributed to his stuttering.

The second means of dealing with problems, intellectualization, is also believed to be problematic in terms of transfer. Another client, whom we'll call Tom, could tell us in great objective detail about stuttering, stuttering theory, speaking events he stuttered in, and the "ways" he stuttered but was next to non-verbal when it came to expressing the attitudes, feelings and emotions that contributed to his stuttering. Instead, he'd concentrate on the way his feet were planted when he spoke or the way the listener was or wasn't postured or dressed rather than what we thought was one of his more primary concerns which was his feeling that ". . . I'll make a fool out of myself if I stutter." Tom would routinely think about his "speech problem" but would rarely act to change it or his contributory beliefs and emotions. In a sense, he was a thinker and not a doer. We need both in this world but if one is going about the serious and difficult business of changing self and then maintaining that change, then he or she needs some of both.

The third way of dealing with problems, projection, is very deleterious, in my opinion, to effective transfer. Here another client, Joe, said that all his listeners, including his speech-language clinician, had particular beliefs, feelings and attitudes; but in reality these "thoughts" were Joe's, not his listener's. He always would give the impression of knowing what his listener was thinking whether the listener said anything or not. He would frequently tell the clinician to stop ". . . treating me like I'm stupid." He would easily and quickly tell how his co-workers had thought this or that about him and how most of his problems were generally the result of evil-thinking and evil-doing on the part of everyone but himself. No amount of talking with Joe convinced him otherwise; nor did psychological counseling, which is, in essence, also "talk-therapy." Interestingly, in the clinic Joe changed his speech behavior to a significant degree, but not his belief that he knew that this or that listener ". . . didn't like me . . . thinks I'm stupid . . . is really inconsiderate." Consequently, he persisted in entering outside-the-clinic communicative situations with the same projecting tendencies (even when he was more fluent) and his fluency slowly but surely eroded in the face of the undermining feelings he ascribed to others. Although acting does impact thinking — more on this later — so does thinking impact acting and Joe's continued projecting thought processes were more conducive to stuttering than fluency. His transfer was nil.

A fourth way of coping with problems that we've found problematic in terms of transfer is the mechanism Vaillant calls reaction formation. This is best exemplified, we think, with some of the parents of child stutterers we've treated. Here a parent, whom we'll call Mrs. Harold, professed a great deal of love and admiration for her child while in our opinion, she actually felt quite differently toward her youngster. Mrs. Harold was all over her son: over-protective, over-nurturing, over-talkative, and over-cautious. Instead of the child's developing some healthy experiences with independence and making a few mistakes, Mrs. Harold kept smothering the child to such a degree that the child seemed to be quite dependent upon her. Consequently, the child would not let the mother out of his sight, refused to participate in therapy to the degree necessary unless the mother was "the therapist." The child was less than willing to cooperate with therapy. The mother's behavior towards her child resulted in exactly what she seemingly didn't want: an overly dependent, uncooperative little boy who didn't allow his mother one moment's solitude. Transfer can't occur until therapy at least starts. Mrs. Harold's means of coping with her feelings towards her son made initiation of therapy very difficult.

Converse to these problematic adjustment mechanisms, are two other means of adapting to problems which Vaillant discusses and which we've found to be indicative of lasting change, that is, effective transfer: (1) altruism and (2) sublimation. Other means of adjustment may also be helpful to transfer, but these two are the ones we have witnessed as being most highly related to transfer. Let me examine them through some case studies.

Altruism happens when an "experienced" stutterer wants to help the "less experienced" stutterer. One client, Ellen, made very nice transfer of her changed speaking and attitudes as she began to set up and run a local self-help group for other adult stutterers. Ellen seemed to really enjoy helping others explore their beliefs and feelings as well as practice changing their speech. She received no extrinsic reward beside the self-satisfaction we believe we all experience when helping others to help themselves really begins to bear fruit. Her setting-up and running of this group were obviously very gratifying to her, and the group, of course, brought her the vicarious satisfaction of watching others succeed. However, her behavior was quite constructive and was reflected back to her in the form of the support she received from those she had helped.

A second means of coping with problems, sublimation, occurs when a stutterer begins to use hobbies, activities, sports, projects, etc., to channel his feelings towards himself and others in constructive, socially acceptable ways. Rather than "drink feelings of anger over stuttering under the table," the stutterer expresses them through achievement of some goal. Although this can be readily seen with some teenagers or adults who stutter, let us examine a parent, Mr. Smith I'll call him, who sublimated his concerns regarding his son into a constructive activity: coaching youth league baseball. Mr. Smith, a big, rugged athletic type, was continually critical of his son, Brian, in terms of Brian's speech, personal habits, and so forth. It was obvious that Brian's rather slight physical build and not overly athletic tendencies were a concern to Mr. Smith. Brian would become fluent in the clinic but Mr. Smith would repeatedly say, ". . . therapy isn't working . . . Brian still stutters at home . . . he just isn't getting any better." It's hard to get cement to dry when you keep pouring water on it! We started to encourage the father to play catch with Brian on a weekly basis and as the weather warmed, to go outside with a bat and ball. With a little more encouragement, the father enrolled Brian in Little League and volunteered to be an assistant coach. We continually harped on the father about the gradualness of change and learning and how Brian would need time and encouragement and fatherly patience to learn baseball. In the meantime, the father became increasingly involved in the team and encouraged not only his son but others as well. Two years from the beginning of this sequence of events, Brian's speech started to stay changed outside as well as inside therapy. Mr. Smith channelled his concerns into constructive social activity from which he, his son, and others benefitted. Brian's transfer was remarkable and an initially very difficult case had a very nice outcome.

While the specific number and nature of variables which impact transfer may differ from one stutterer to another, variables such as those discussed above appear to warrant careful consideration prior to and during therapy. We should recognize that transfer, particularly the lack thereof, of fluent speech is not always the result of the therapy program. It may also be a result of the type of client who enters the therapy room. Given the above discussion, let us briefly examine the four types of clients we believe enter stuttering therapy — the dissatisfied, the satisfied, the dreamers and the changers — and see how each might be expected to transfer.

Transfer: The Dreamers, The Dissatisfied, The Satisfied and The Changers

1. The Dreamers. We seem to have most of our transfer problems with those stutterers who have made the decision to change but not the conscious commitment to engage in the activities necessary to realize such change. We term these clients the "dreamers" because they dream of change but shun the realities of making and transferring that change. They are the clients who find the effort not worth the cost and who seem to routinely "forget" therapy outside the clinic. Their decision to change makes them at least willing to "be cured" in the clinic but outside the clinic, where they must take a very active, "doing" role in maintaining that change, they run into problems. Somehow, some way the speech-language clinician has to convince these "dreaming" clients that change is an ongoing, extra-clinical endeavor. Clinicians must explain and re-explain that change in speech and related beliefs/emotions is an activity that only **begins** in the clinic, and that for it to last, it must be continued into the client's everyday life. Surely the client's insights into himself and his behavior derived from our therapies are of help; however, he must **act** on these insights inside, but more importantly, outside the clinic. Transfer is indeed difficult for the client who is really not willing and able to be an active participant in the process of change. This doesn't mean he or she is a bad person, only a human one. After all, if changing our more undesirable characteristics was an easy task we'd all be Goody Twoshoes.

2. The Dissatisfied. Of even greater difficulty, in terms of transfer, are the clients who are not interested in changing even though dissatisfied with speech and self. We term these clients "dissatisfied" and find them the poorest bet in terms of change/ transfer of change. We might ask ourselves how we **make** someone who doesn't want to change decide to change that which they don't like about themselves? Surely, we must not overstate the case to such clients in terms of their speech and related problems but neither must we down-play it. Objective information delivered in firm but supportive tones may help some of these people decide to change and commit themselves to the actions necessary to realize such change; however, some will still be unwilling to change despite their dissatisfaction. This is particularly difficult with the older child, teenager and adult who do not like the way they talk but who are familiar with their speech and reluctant to make the necessary commitment to change. Some of these clients seem to hope against hope that "it" will go away with time. The fact that stuttering does not disappear with time may help some of the "dissatisfied" decide to commit themselves to change.

3. The Satisfied. A third group, generally the very young child who stutters, is actually "satisfied" with his or her speech and self. In fact, the young child who is not dissatisfied is probably the rule rather than the exception. With these young children, behavioral change on the part of the child as well as, where appropriate, parental attitude change, will probably be sufficient for effective transfer. This is particularly true if the child is not "locked" into fluency-inhibiting behavior and attitudes and the parents are capable of changing their own communicative and related attitudes.

4. The Changers. The fourth group, the changers, are the clinician's success stories. They change in the clinic and effectively transfer this change into their everyday lives. Perhaps their speech and related behaviors are not as habituated and associated with concomitant problems, such as, articulation problems (Cullinan and Springer), or developmental delays in neuromotor processes for speech production. Whatever it may be, they transfer. Perhaps the key to the motivation of the "changers" is a caring and capable-of-changing mother/father or their desire to give a good job interview or their interest in moving up the career ladder, or their desire to meet members of the opposite sex more easily. Maybe their adjustment to problems, for example, use of sublimation, gives them positive, facilitatory means to change. We still don't know why such people change and transfer but this group of clients definitely deserve careful, objective appraisal. We may not be able to bottle what they "have" but at least we would be better able to recognize them and adjust our prognosis accordingly.

Transfer: Ideal versus Real

Thorndike said that transfer depends upon the presence of identical elements, either in content or procedure, in the original learning and the new learning situation. In other words, the more the clinic and environment have in common (the more they "overlap") in terms of content and procedure, the higher the probability that that which is learned in the clinic will be transferred to the environment. In terms of transfer the successful clinic, according to Thorndike, and common sense, will have much of the environment within it. For the stutterer, of course, one of the most important environments, is that housed within him or herself. Although the clinic can try to motivate the stutterer to change and attempt to create a realistic situation in which the client tries out his "new" speech, it should be apparent that ultimately it is up to the stutterer to change.

Williams states that ". . . the essence of stuttering therapy is the transfer and maintenance of a desired response pattern; obtaining fluency is not the major goal." This statement, we believe, sums up very nicely why our therapies with stutterers so often result in less than optimal transfer; that is, too much of our therapy time is spent achieving within-clinic change and too little time is spent working on outside-of-clinic realities. The realities we speak of here are those of trying to remember to produce new behaviors — physiological as well as psychological — in emotionally and communicatively difficult speaking situations. It's hard to remember "your new speech" in speaking situations that conjure up fears, attitudes and remembrances of past failures or difficulties. We may be able to teach the actual act of fluency but unless it is performed simultaneously with changed attitudinal/emotional responses, the stutterer's fluency will quickly deteriorate and transfer will be minimal, at least in the long run.

In attempts to show how such common elements might actually work in therapy, we will present a case study which my doctoral student, Howard D. Schwartz, and myself have been doing what we'll term experimental therapy. Simply put, we are "feeding back" to the client, as he is talking, information about his laryngeal behavior by means of an electroglottograph, (Fourcin; Rothenberg) that appears facilitory as well as inhibitory to his fluency.

We believe that such therapy has common elements, at least in terms of speech production, with the client's outside-of-clinic speaking because we are helping him help himself **feel** (not listen, see, or taste) what he is **doing** that is helping or hindering his speech **as** he is speaking. Not **after** he has spoken but **during** the actual instances in time when he is interfering with the forward flow of his speech. These feelings of inap-

23

propriate tensions and postures of, in this case, laryngeal events, are common to his speech both inside and outside the clinic. This client's ability to quickly, accurately and objectively identify that which he is doing that needs change is believed by us to be of major benefit to him in learning how to change these behaviors and to keep them changed.

We should note that this young person was chosen as our first client to systematically employ these procedures with because he had: (1) received but failed with previous therapies, (2) appeared to have little objective awareness of his speech behavior and (3) possessed the willingness and ability to discuss attitudes, beliefs and fears that may contribute to his stuttering. That is, while we wanted a client whose lack of objective awareness of the **physical feelings** of speech production made our feedback procedures most appropriate, we also wanted a client who could deal with the non-physiological aspects as well. After about 10 sessions with us the young man has improved his ability to recognize and change his inappropriate speech behavior. He has also become increasingly able to recognize attitudes which stand in his way when making these changes in his speech outside the clinic. It is, however, a long rough road. It is also very clear that he will be able to make the changes in his speech physiology long before he makes the changes in his attitudes. Changes in his speech do help him change his attitudes or at least make some of these changes easier to make, but without changes in his concerns about speaking, he will not be able to transfer the type of speech production necessary to speak fluently outside the clinic.

This case study points up the need, as Williams and others (for example, Boberg) have done, to both (1) change speech behaviors and attitudes as well as (2) incorporate transfer within therapy. The feedback procedures we are using and developing help the client quickly and correctly "feel" (not hear or see) what he is doing that helps or hinders fluency and thus, we hope, transfer these feelings into real world speaking situations. One must, of course, continually remind the client that such procedures, such "gadgets" as the electroglottograph (Fourcin; Rothenberg) which we used, are merely means to an end. The client must use them as a training device, as a means of accurately and objectively focusing his attention on behavior. The client should not be encouraged to use them like eyeglasses which are, of course, a permanent means of correcting a problem.

The client, at the same time, definitely needs time to explore beliefs and feelings that contribute to the problem. If these feelings and beliefs are ignored, particularly with the older client, the clinician does so at the risk of winning the battle but losing the war. The stutterer not only acts, he or she also thinks. As we've discussed elsewhere (Conture), the two intertwine in their influence on the person and his or her behavior. We are convinced that the high incidence of relapse for many human problems — smoking, depression, drinking and so forth — is due to the fact that either the clinician is either too behavioristic **or** too mentalistic. The stutterer, just like the normally fluent speaker, does not live by feelings **or** behavior alone. He thinks and he behaves, he behaves and he thinks. The two can be separated, for sake of clinical expedience, pedagogical description or philosophical persuasions, but to do so continually in the clinic is to achieve short-term gain at the risk of engendering long-term pain when the client's problem relapses to its before-therapy state.

Because the stutterer behaves and some of this behavior "gets in the way" of his fluency, it behooves the stutterer to "think" about how he is behaving. However, we believe along with others that not just any type of "thinking" will do (for example, Van Riper). This is particularly true with regard to transfer. The stutterer, to get the most lasting behavioral change, **must feel what it is that he is doing** that facilitates or inhibits his fluency. Feeling here does not mean emoting but actually sensing the right and wrong physiology (tensions, postures and movements) necessary to produce fluent speech. Simply put, lasting behavioral change requires quick, accurate and objective feeling/sensing of inhibitory speech physiology. Likewise, lasting attitudinal changes, changes without which fluency will not transfer, require the stutterer to recognize and react differently to external/ internal environmental stimuli (Williams). Achieving such attitudinal changes requires "talk therapy" during which the client explores those attitudes, beliefs, fears, and emotions which lead him to react to certain stimuli with fluency-inhibiting emotions. Not easy but who ever said it would be?

Many times, particularly with youngsters under 10 years of age, the clinician may want and need to deal with the parents' attitudes. It is quite possible that transfer with the young child is directly related to the degree to which parents change their attitudes and beliefs which appear contributory to the child's stuttering. And some parents, just like some stutterers, are quite resistive to changing their own ideas, attitudes, and beliefs, particularly if they believe these changes will make them change their standards for child rearing and discipline. We have found that the best approach with such parents is not to tell them how harmful their beliefs or standards are but to make them quite aware of the fact that changing their behavior will positively change their child's behavior. Don't look, of course, for rapid change in these situations but do persist in helping parents modify their non-facilitatory child-parent interactions.

It should be evident from the above that establishment of behavior change comes rather quickly, particularly with therapies that directly manipulate the stutterer's speech production. Transfer of this behavioral change, however, often fades out as quickly as it was established. Paradoxically, establishment of attitudinal/belief system changes takes quite some time but once these changes are made they seem to transfer to outside-the-clinic fairly readily. Perhaps, there is a lesson here. Quick, in-clinic change of speech or attitudes may be obtained at the risk of poor transfer of this change to outside the clinic. Maybe there is a fixed period of time that must transpire before any change in ourself or our behavior can be truly transferable into the environment.

As mentioned above it is now popular to talk about "...working on transfer from the beginning of therapy"; however, if we are really going to work on transfer right from the beginning of therapy, we should be honest with our clients in terms of the time, effort and sacrifice this procedure will take. The time issue is one that is of particular concern. Too often the length of our therapy regimen is dictated by the inappropriate time schedules of others, that is, the public-school calendar, the employer's need to have the employee "fluent in two months," the university senior's need in March to be "fluent before I graduate in May," and so forth. How can transfer take place when true establishment of behavioral change hasn't occurred? We must communicate our legitimate concerns to our clients regarding these time restrictions. If we don't, who will?

References

Barron, F., "Personal Soundness in University Graduate Students" in *Creativity and Psychological Health.* Princeton: O. Van Nostrand Company, 1963.

Boberg, E. (Ed.), *Maintenance of Fluency.* New York: Lemcke and Buechner, 1981.

Buscaglia, L., *Love.* New York: Fawcett Crest, 1982.

Cahn, S., "The Art of Teaching" in *American Educator,* 6, 36-39, 1982.

Conture, E., *Stuttering.* Englewood Cliffs, NJ: Prentice-Hall, 1982.

Cullinan, W., and Springer, M., "Voice Initiation and Termination Times in Stuttering and Non-stuttering Children" in *Journal of Speech and Hearing Research,* 23, 344-360, 1980.

Fourcin, A., "Laryngographic Assessment of Phonatory Function," in Ludlow, C. and Hart, M. (Eds.), *Proceedings of the Conference on the Assessment of Vocal Pathology. ASHA Reports 11.* Danville, IL: Interstate Printers, Inc., 1982.

Mencken, H. L., *A Mencken Chrestomathy.* New York: Vintage Books, 1982.

Rothenberg, M., "Some Relations Between Glottal Air Flow and Vocal Fold Contact Area" in Ludlow, C. and Hart, M. (Eds.), *Proceedings of the Conference on the Assessment of Vocal Pathology., ASHA Reports 11.* Danville, IL: Interstate Printers, Inc., 1982.

Thorndike, E. L., *Educational Psychology.* New York: Lemcke and Buechner, 1903.

Vaillant, G., *Adaptation to Life.* Boston: Little, Brown and Company, 1977.

Van Riper, C., *The Treatment of Stuttering.* Englewood Cliffs, NJ: Prentice-Hall, Inc., 1973.

Williams, D. E., "A Perspective on Approaches to Stuttering Therapy" in Gregory, H. (Ed.), *Controversies About Stuttering Therapy.* Baltimore: University Park Press, 1978.

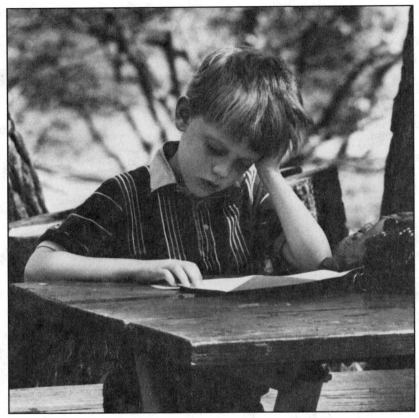

chapter two

Working with Children in the School Environment

by Dean E. Williams, Ph.D.

The purpose of this chapter is to discuss ways to accomplish — and some problems involved in — "transfer" and "maintenance" in stuttering therapy for elementary school aged children. Ordinarily the clinician works to "establish" a desired response pattern in the therapy room and then to transfer it to outside situations. Problems can and do arise when clinicians consider that they are generalizing a speech pattern that has already been learned. This "has learned" viewpoint too often reflects the faulty assumption that the child has learned a speech production skill in the therapy room and that the transfer phase involves only habitually "using" the learned behavior in outside situations. Instead, when a child leaves the therapy room and talks to a friend or to his teacher he is not solely transferring a response pattern, he also is **establishing** a new reaction pattern. The communicative interaction changed from the one that existed in the therapy room.

Stuttering develops as a communication problem every bit as much, if not more so, as it does a speech production problem. The essence of therapy is to help the child cope constructively with his speech production abilities in the presence of the feelings involved in his ever-changing communicative interactions. From this perspective, the concepts of "transfer and maintenance" — if considered to encompass solely speech production skills — can be misleading to the beginning clinician. We hope to clarify this point in the following discussion.

As stuttering develops in children their feelings become a fundamental part of **their** stuttering, and by so doing, stuttering becomes part of **them.** This is one reason that for many children, their stuttering is so personal — and so private. To them, their feelings represent the internal part of their stutter. The speaking behavior that the listener observes, is the part that the child could not hide. Various terms have been used to discuss these "stuttering feelings," for example, anxiety, anticipation, stress, negative emotion, fear, etc., etc. Regardless of the terms used, most theorists agree that a person's "feelings" become paired with the overt struggle behaviors. Hence, a change in a person's feelings may trigger an instance of stuttering. These "feelings of stuttering" result from a combination of emotional and motoric feelings. They combine to serve as internal cues that the child comes to monitor before or as he speaks in order, he hopes, to be better able to cope with the ways he talks.

We are well aware that our emotional feelings change constantly as we talk to different people, in different places, in different roles, about different topics, with different language structures, etc. As a result, the internal cues that the child experiences are changing constantly. Therefore, to rephrase what I stated earlier: a clinician's task, fundamentally, is to help the child **learn how to learn** to cope constructively with changing communicative interactions and the internal cues that are such a vital part of them.

In the discussion that follows, the term "transfer" refers **not** to a response that has been learned but rather to the transferring — establishing process involved in learning to cope with differing communicative environments. Furthermore, my comments will focus on those issues commonly found in the elementary school environment.

The therapy program that the clinician develops in a school system should take into account the unique aspects of each school in which she works. She will need to explain to the principal, teacher, etc., the structure of the stuttering therapy program so that she, with the help of these school personnel, can work together to adapt, where possible, school policies and regulations to fit her therapy program. The three main aspects of structuring a program are (1) the frequency and length of therapy sessions per week, (2) the support by and cooperation of the school personnel for the child and for the therapy program, and (3) the clinical procedures used during the therapy sessions that will promote their use in the school environment.

Scheduling Therapy Sessions

The clinician should schedule therapy sessions frequently enough per week and of sufficient duration to meet the needs of the child who stutters. To attempt to force a stutterer into an established "school schedule" — for example, of two 15 minute individual sessions per week — is being professionally irresponsible. A school clinician must adapt her schedule to fit the needs of the client. If this cannot be done, the child should be referred to someone who can. Ordinarily two to three individual sessions per week, each for 30-40 minutes, is a **minimal** requirement. In addition, however, the clinician should plan on time to be spent with school personnel and, if possible, the child's parents. This may appear to be a great deal of time to spend with one client in the schools but (1) the nature of the stuttering problem requires more clinician time than some of the other speech problems do, and (2) most clinicians who spend less time than this report very little success with the stuttering child.

Preparing the Environment for Transfer

In order for a child to transfer improved speech into his school environment, he is required to begin behaving in ways that are different from the ways he has behaved in the past. For many children, this can be rather frightening. They are unsure of what they will do and how other people will react. For them, when they act in ways in which they are not used to acting they feel conspicuous. They feel "strange" or "kind of funny." They are afraid that people will notice — and say something! As a result, it is not uncommon for stuttering children to prefer to act "like themselves" and to just hope that they do not stutter. In my experience, it often has been difficult for clinicians to realize that for many children, it is more important at times to communicate their thoughts and their feelings "honestly" than it is to say the words fluently.

Obviously, it is easier for a child to change certain ways of acting and to observe the consequences if the people in his environment are supportive and reinforcing to the ways he is communicating — both verbally and nonverbally. These people, teachers, principals, etc., can be important contributors to a child's successful transfer — and maintenance — of improved fluency.

When a clinician accepts a child who stutters for therapy in a school, it is important for her to open lines of communication with the principal and the child's classroom teacher. In discussions with them, the clinician can find out how they "see" the child. What do they like about the ways he acts, both verbally and nonverbally, and what things do they dislike — and wish he could change? When the child stutters, what bothers them the most about it? Is it for example, when he tenses so much, or when he holds his breath, or when he keeps looking at the floor? The information obtained can be used at a later date in discussion with teachers and principals. The clinician may want to work with the child to change certain ways he acts (verbally or nonverbally) that his teacher, for example, did not like. Then, the clinician can alert her to notice the change and to comment upon it. This can help the child learn to feel free to change the ways he acts.

The nature of stuttering should be discussed with the principal and the teacher. They need to understand the relation of communicative interaction to the problem and the need to modify these interactions as a part of therapy. In this way they can obtain a perspective about what therapy involves and ways that they can be helpful. For example, several years ago, we had a conference with a group of principals and teachers who had stutterers in their schools. We asked them if they talked to the stutterers informally in the halls or between classes as much as they did to children who do not stutter. Their answer was "no." When we discussed the reasons for this, several of them verbalized, and others agreed, that it honestly was not because they were embarrassed when the child stuttered. After all, they were used to working with children with problems. Rather, it was because if they talked to the child and the child stuttered in answering, they felt responsible for making the child stutter. It was "their" fault if he stuttered. They believed they were being kind by not placing the child in the turmoil of having to talk and to stutter. This example is used to point out the kinds of misconceptions that exist. Principals and teachers want to help children. It is the clinician's responsibility to help them learn ways to do it.

The principal needs to be provided with information about the structure of the clinician's therapy program. Then he will understand the logic behind requests to take the child into the halls during class time even though it is ordinarily against school policy. He is more likely to permit this so that the clinician and the child can talk to the janitor, the cook, the secretary — and even to him.

The classroom teacher needs to understand the therapy program so that she can understand her place in it. It is especially important that the clinician work for open lines of communication with the teacher based on mutual sensitivity and understanding. In talking to groups of school clinicians, the most common complaint I hear is that the classroom teacher is "not cooperative." This is unfortunate. It is difficult for me to believe that a teacher who is devoting her professional life to helping children will refuse to help children. After discussions with many classroom teachers, a different picture emerges from that reported by the clinicians. Some report that they do not understand what they can do to be helpful, and why it will help, as opposed to doing something else. Also, they resent, at times, the way they are "told" what to do. The clinician comes to her room, tells her that she is doing this and this wrong and that she should be doing this — then leaves. Other complaints involve the problem of time. When a teacher has thirty and even forty children in a class, it is unreasonable to expect her to spend undue time with one child at the expense of the others. Other problems of time occur that reflect a lack of understanding or sensitivity on the part of the clinician. For example, the clinician bursts in on the teacher to have a conference when the teacher has ten minutes to make final preparations for the remainder of the day.

The other major complaint involves requests by clinicians that are unreasonable. Several examples will illustrate the point. One clinician informed the teacher that Johnny was learning to "stutter smoothly." She requested the teacher to stop Johnny anytime he did not "stutter smoothly" and make him do it again until it was "smooth." One might argue about the advisability of using such procedures; however, a more critical issue is the fact that the teacher was not trained — and had no way of knowing — how "smooth" stuttering has to be before it is "smooth enough?" The other example concerns a clinician who was attempting to transfer to the classroom the fluency the child had learned in the therapy room. She requested that for the first week the teacher ask the child questions that could be answered with only three words. The next week the questions were to be answered with only five words. Teachers cannot be expected to serve as surrogate clinicians. The clinician should assume the responsibility for blending the therapy activities into the daily classroom routine.

The clinician can discuss with the teacher the daily activities that occur with the children. She should learn about the various opportunities that the children have to speak each day. Do they have a chance to answer questions, to ask them, to tell a story, to read aloud, etc.? How does "Chester" do in these activities? In which does he appear to have the most difficulty — the least? The clinician should determine also the types of materials and books used with each subject taught and then utilize them where possible in therapy. In preparing the child to transfer improved speech into the classroom, the clinician can incorporate a reality into the therapy room activities that the child can understand.

The teacher can be asked about the ways that it would be most convenient for her to communicate with the clinician about the child's needs. This may be done, for example, by any combination of the following: write short notes; establish a specific time during a day, e.g., recess or gym time, when the teacher is "more likely" to have free time; eat lunch together on days when you have information to share; or make phone calls at home. Obviously, there are many other ways it can be done. The point is that mutual sharing of decisions enhances the opportunities for cooperation.

The clinician can discuss with the teacher ways that she would feel comfortable participating in the therapy program. Her role will vary from situation to situation. Generally, the teacher can be extremely helpful by being supportive of the changes the child is making. She can provide the opportunities for the child to speak and she can observe his performance. She **should not be** expected to directly "correct" or "modify" the child's speech. In fact, she should refrain from doing so — one clinician is enough.

In my opinion, one of the most important ways that the teacher can assist in the transfer aspect of therapy for a child is through her supportive role as "his teacher." Prior to asking the child to practice improved ways of talking in the classroom, it should be demonstrated to the teacher. Some teachers are able to visit the therapy room and observe just what it is the child is practicing. Others will meet with the child and the clinician in the classroom after school. In this way, the teacher will know what to expect. More importantly, now the child knows that the teacher knows — and that she approves. Furthermore, now the clinician and the teacher stand side by side in what they **expect** the child to do and this makes it easier for the child to be successful. Also, it opens up communication between the teacher and the child about his therapy program.

The clinician's interactions with the parents of the child can be similar to those with the teacher. There needs to be a discussion in order for them to understand the therapy program and their place in it. Also, prior to the time when the child is to transfer improved ways of talking to the home environment, one or both of the parents should, if at all possible, join the clinician and the child so that they can demonstrate for the parent(s) the changes he is making. Again, as with his teacher, he now knows that they know what to expect — and that his mother and/or father approve. During the course of the therapy program, much of the communication between the clinician and the parents can be done by phone.

Preparing the Child for the Transfer of Improved Speech

The clinician cannot take the responsibility for "ensuring success" outside of the clinic room. The child must do it. The clinician does have the obligation, however, to maximize the chances that the child will be able to cope constructively with his communicative interactions involving increased emotion.

One must realize that it takes courage as well as motivation for a person to change his behavior. Furthermore, it takes courage — and for some, a great deal of courage — to change speaking behavior in prescribed ways when he is scared of what might occur and fearful that he might fail. A child is no different from anyone else.

A clinician can talk with the child. She can find out his beliefs about stuttering. What does he think is wrong with him? Why does he stutter? What does he do to help himself talk "better?" What would he do or what would it sound like if he did not do that to "help himself?" How does he feel when he stutters? What does he think other people think of him when he stutters? These, as well as other questions, can be discussed with the child using language and examples that can be understood and shared. This can serve as the foundation from which to discuss with him what is "going on" when he stutters — the things he can do that will make it harder to talk — the things he can do to help. From this, the clinician can discuss the therapy program. This should include what he will be asked to do, why he will do it, and what he will accomplish. The child should be made to feel that he is a participant in his own therapy program. Also, she can discuss with him his confusions and his fears about stuttering. He should be helped to understand that his "bad" feelings are normal — that he is "normal," he is "okay" — that he can learn to talk acceptably — that he will goof at times but that he can do it — and, that the clinician, teacher, and parents are there to help in any way he wants them to help. When a child knows what is wrong, when he understands what he can do to help, when he feels relatively good about himself, and when he realizes people are supportive, it is much easier to have courage than it is when his talking world is mysterious, confusing and lonely.

In the therapy room, the clinician ordinarily works with the child in order to establish a desired speech response pattern. The "desired" behavior will vary from clinician to clinician depending upon her approach to therapy. Regardless of the approach used, however, the difficulty of establishing a desired response pattern usually will increase with increased complexity of the speaking interactions. These include the **social complexity,** the **language-propositionality complexity,** and the **reaction complexity.**

The social complexity involves those speaking situations usually thought of as the "transfer stage." They include, for example: talking to the clinician alone in the therapy room; talking to another child or an adult in the hall; talking to the teacher; and talking in the classroom.

The language-propositionality complexity refers to the nature of the speaking task. It involves, for example, the following: a one word response; a short comment; asking a question; answering a question; reading a word, sentence or a paragraph; telling a story or a joke; describing an event; and discussing opinions. Each of the above represents a different speaking task. There are, of course, many more.

The reaction complexity refers either to the way the listener reacts to the speaker or the way the speaker reacts to the speaking task. The listener may, for example, be attentive, be distracted and be paying little attention to what is said, be irritated and hurried, be smiling or chuckling, or be disgusted and shake his head and frown. On the other hand, the speaker may react and speak rapidly, slowly, hurriedly, deliberately, excitedly, calmly, etc. As each of the reactions of the speaker and listener change, the communicative interaction changes. The clinician can help the child learn to cope constructively with these changing listener reactions.

The child can practice the desired manner of speaking in the therapy room with the clinician. This first will be done at one level of language-propositionality complexity, with the clinician reacting with a constant level of complexity, usually attentively and calmly. Then, the child can vary the language-propositionality complexity. Also, the clinician can vary the listener's reaction pattern by role playing different reactions. Together, they can note the ways the child's feelings and speaking behavior change. This can help the child prepare for speaking outside of the therapy room. It can serve to emphasize the need to practice in "easy situations" in order to know what to do at those times when increased emotion is involved.

The clinician can then vary systematically the complexity of the speaking situation. The child first practices with the clinician. Then, prior to entering an outside situation, for example, asking the teacher a question, the clinician and child can role play the situation. The clinician is "the teacher" and the child asks the desired question. This is practiced until the child feels that he knows what to do. Then, he can go and ask his teacher the question. This type of therapy structure can be followed for increasingly complex speaking situations.

Children differ in the ease with which they transfer the improved manner of speaking. Some are able to transfer easily and consistently into increasingly difficult situations following a period of role playing with the clinician. Others have more difficulty. They are those with relatively strong emotional reactions associated with talking and stuttering. For these, it is helpful for the clinician to accompany the child during the early stages of transfer. For some, this is all that is needed. For others, more is needed. For these children, the clinician can help the child verbalize and accept his feelings of fear. For example, just before entering the situation, the clinician can say "are you scared now? Do you feel real funny right in your stomach? It's okay to be scared. Feel it. It doesn't hurt you. You can still talk even though you are scared. Let's practice again saying what you plan to say while you are scared. Good. Good. I'm with you. Let's go in and you begin to talk the way you want to — even though you are scared." Once a child learns that he can cope constructively with his feelings and the way he talks, transfer progresses rapidly. School personnel can be very helpful. For example, the teacher can talk with the child about ways she can help. The school secretary, the janitor and the cook can help by encouraging him to keep up the good work. Successful transfer into the school environment provides a firm foundation for maintenance of his improved speech.

Maintaining Improved Fluency

Early in this paper the point was made that the child is continually "establishing" improved fluency as he enters new situations. A therapy program should prepare him for such a challenge. This same concept exists for what is commonly called the "maintenance program." Maintenance involves no more than continuing the transfer phase, which in turn, involves no more than expanding the "establishing phase." We are dealing with a continuing **process**. We separate, at times, the learning process into three "phases" or "categories" for convenience of discussion and not because they reflect the reality of behavior change and stabilization.

In my opinion, if the child understands what he is doing to talk the ways he wants to talk, if he understands that he is continually learning to improve his speech, and if he understands that in learning we all "goof" at times, then he will be able to cope constructively with times when he occasionally stutters. If he does not understand these things, then, following an instance of stuttering, he will be prepared for little more than to "hope" that he will not do it again. This can rekindle feelings of fear and of helplessness. These feelings can be one of the first steps leading to regression.

As the child is transferring improved fluency into more and more types of verbal interactions, the clinician can be laying the foundation for maintaining this improvement. The child can participate in the planning of speaking tasks. This can lead to a period of time when he will make and carry out the assignments. The clinician's task is to help him learn meaningful ways to do it and to assess **with him** his progress. As a child becomes competent at planning, carrying out, and assessing his own daily speaking activities, then the clinician can begin stretching out times between clinical sessions. She may begin to meet with the child every two or three weeks. Then, if successful, the time period can be extended. If the child begins to experience difficulties in coping, they can meet more often until he gets back "on track." Then, the time periods can be extended again.

There are advantages to continuing to meet with the child for a year every two to three weeks even for 15 minutes each time. This helps him learn that therapy is not "ended." It emphasizes the fact that he is "expected" to continue improving. Furthermore, it provides for him the opportunity of having someone to "answer to" and having someone who can share his speaking experiences. In addition to this type of program, the school environment offers the opportunity to obtain the evaluations of other persons. The clinician can check with the teacher, secretary, principal, etc., who talk with the child. She can go out of her way to meet the child in the hall to ask, "How is it going?"

If he says "okay," a smile, a wink, a pat on the back can keep things active and rewarding.

Embodied in the short talks with the child over time can be the philosophy that he is a pretty "normal kid" who may get tangled up at times when he talks — but that if he does, **he can change what he is doing** and talk the ways he wants to talk.

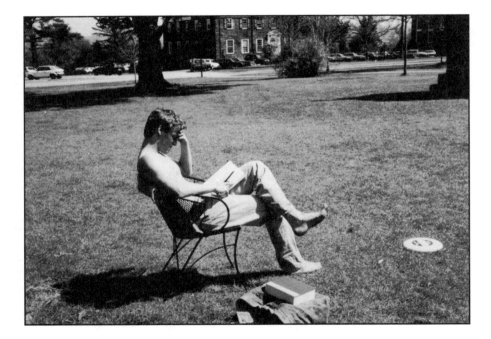

chapter three

Behavioral Transfer and Maintenance Programs for Adolescent and Adult Stutterers

by Einer Boberg, Ph.D.

In this paper I will describe our transfer and maintenance programs for adult and adolescent stutterers. To help explain the rationale and strategies used in the transfer and maintenance phases I will provide a brief outline of the initial phases of treatment in which we train clients in self-identification, teach prolongation and other fluency skills and establish normal sounding speech within the clinic. The rationale and procedures used in the establishment phases of the program lead directly into the clinical procedures used in the transfer and maintenance phases.

Establishment Program and Preparation for Transfer

In our intensive residential program clients meet 7 hours/day for 3 weeks. Clients are selected on a first-come basis rather than according to severity. Groups range in size from four to six and provide a natural setting in which clients develop conversational and interpersonal skills while progressing through systematic modifications of their speech. Audio and video recordings are made of their pre and post-clinic speech in a variety of settings including reading single words, sentences, text, conversing with strangers, talking on the telephone and talking to the clinician. All pre and post-tapes are analyzed with the assistance of electronic equipment. This equipment is a system of counters and timers arranged in such a way that the clinician, using two microswitches, can count all stuttered and non-stuttered syllables within a unit of time. These data are converted to percentage of syllables stuttered and syllable rate per minute. The equipment provides each client immediate individualized feedback while he is talking within the group setting. The equipment is used throughout the treatment program to count stuttered and non-stuttered syllables.

The therapy program is organized into several phases. After we have achieved a measure of the client's baserate of stuttering each client learns to identify the occurrence of stuttering behaviors in ongoing speech. In Phase III clients begin to explore how to make various speech sounds without struggle or tension. They learn how to initiate sound with an easy, relaxed manner. We also practice other fluency skills such as correct phrasing and soft contacts on consonants. Next we move into formal prolongation sessions where each client must complete a number of sessions at 60 spm with less than 1% stuttering. When he has reached criterion he takes a self-assessment test and then begins to increase his speech rate systematically until he reaches the rate of 190±20. He also learns to cancel his errors immediately by stopping as soon as he struggles to repeat the stuttered word several times. He monitors his own speech and uses a variable speech rate. During the 3 week period, clients spend many hours in group discussions and debating provocative topics. Much discussion revolves around attitudes and experiences common to stutterers. We encourage these discussions to emerge spontaneously as the clients begin to know each other and wish to share their experiences and feelings. The clinician tries to move the discussions from a recital of negative, defeatist attitudes toward an exploration of those attitudes that may be of some benefit in stabilizing the behavior in the post-clinic environment.

We also spend considerable time and effort in fostering a

positive attitude toward transfer in clients. We suggest that they view transfer as an opportunity to try new clinical skills in the outside environment as a chance to "try their wings." Although most clients will succeed in transfer far more than they will fail, we suggest that they welcome difficulties as well as successes. The failed attempts can be used to learn about themselves, to analyze what happened, where they erred, and to plan corrective strategies. Each situation, and particularly those they fear, should be viewed as an opportunity to experiment, to set up a target and to evaluate their performance. When they understand that an error or a sudden reversion to struggle behavior during a transfer assignment does not spell disaster, this realization helps build their self-confidence. We encourage them to realize that as they now approach feared situations they do possess strategies to cope effectively; they know how to recover, make appropriate corrections and learn from the situation.

The following diagram may help the reader to visualize the various phases in the establishment program.

Pre-Clinic Testing
Audio and video samples of speech

↓

Baserate Measures in Group Setting

↓

Identification
Clients learn to identify and describe stuttering behavior

↓

Preparation for Prolongation
Speech mechanism is described
Fluency skills are introduced

↓

Prolongation
Fluency skills stabilized
Self assessment
Clinic visitor program

↓

Systematic Rate Increase
Cancellation procedures are taught
Corrective rate changes are practiced
Attitudes and experiences are discussed

↓

Self-Monitoring and Transfer Training

↓

Transfer Activities

↓

Post-Clinic Testing
Same as in pre-clinic testing

↓

Maintenance Program
Home activities
Clinic visits
Speech evaluations

Additional information about this program and related programs is available in other publications listed at the end of this chapter.

When clients can produce normal sounding speech at normal rates with less than 1% disfluency within the clinic, they are ready to move into the transfer phase of the program.

Recording and Analysis of Transfer Assignments

In preparation for transfer, clients are asked to purchase a portable cassette recorder equipped with a tape counter, a remote hand-held microphone with off/on switch or a pause button so that they can easily switch off the recorder when the audience speaks. We tape record all transfer activities. Cassette recorders can be used overtly or covertly. We rejected the latter for a variety of reasons including practical and ethical ones. That left the option of carrying the recorder and explaining to the audience that he, the client, was enrolled in a therapy course and was required to tape his conversation so that he could analyze it afterwards. We have seldom encountered any reluctance on the part of the audience to participate, particularly when they understand that their portion of the conversation will not be recorded.

During transfer we use the same format as in the establishment period where a session is defined as the completion of five minutes of talking time for each client. In order to complete one transfer session each client must enter situations until he has accumulated five minutes of talk-time.

Each client is responsible for completing the transfer session and analyzing the tape before he hands it to the clinician for evaluation. The client must note which words are disfluent, which words were cancelled correctly, what aspects need to be improved and whether he was employing fluency skills such as correct phrasing, rate, continuity of airflow, prosody, soft contacts and easy onsets. Moreover, the tape must contain a minimum of five minutes of speech spoken at normal rates with less than 2% disfluency. When he has analyzed his tape the client completes an analysis form and then compares his evaluation with a similar evaluation made by the clinician when she has heard the tape. The client will be aided considerably in estimating the correct time period for his session if the recorder is equipped with a tape counter.

We have divided the transfer assignments into two groups. There are 12 standard assignments which we ask everyone to complete. These are followed by 10 personalized assignments which are developed around the particular needs of each client.

Standard Transfers

We have arranged the 12 standard assignments in order of presumed difficulty but the client may rearrange the tasks if he wishes.

1. Conversations with secretaries/staff within the clinic building. We start with this situation since it is easier for clients to make the initial transfer in the building where there are many conditioned cues for fluent controlled speech. This low-pressure situation also allows the client to become familiar with the mechanics of recording and timing. In this first transfer situation we ask the client to include several rate changes, alternating from a slow rate of 100 spm to a normal rate of 200 spm.

2-4. Opinion surveys. Since it is difficult for most people to approach strangers and engage in conversation we have adopted a survey format to facilitate and legitimize contacts with strangers. The client approaches a stranger, explains that he is enrolled in a therapy program and requests a few minutes of their time. He then poses a number of questions about stuttering. The nature of the audience response is less important than the opportunity to talk to strangers about stuttering and demonstrate fluency controls to them and to himself. Clients continue in this activity until they have completed three five minute sessions.

5-6. Conversations with strangers.   At this stage we now ask clients to engage strangers in conversation without the comforting props of the previous step. Our clinic happens to be across the street from a psychiatric walk-in clinic and we have been able to work out an arrangement to our mutual satisfaction. The important thing is to have the clients approach strangers, initiate and maintain a conversation using controlled fluency and produce a clinically acceptable tape recording of the conversation.

7-8. Telephone assignments.   In the next two assignments clients make calls to commercial firms listed in the yellow pages or the classified ads of the local paper. Clients are to record only their own portion of the conversation. It will usually be necessary to make several phone calls in order to complete one 5 minute assignment.

9-11. Shopping assignments.   In these assignments clients are asked to enter situations in which they might have extended conversations such as shopping for a car, major appliances, vacation travels, real estate, etc. We suggest that they always inform the merchant about the tape recorder and then if he objects they should thank him and leave. In our experience most merchants do not object and quickly come to ignore the recorder. Some clients express concern about taking up the merchant's time when they have no intention of making a purchase. We point out that normal speakers regularly go shopping without an obligation to buy and that merchants are prepared for this.

12. Job interview.   As the final assignment of the standard transfer we require that each client schedule and complete a job interview. We suggest that these interviews be arranged in areas of genuine interest or within their current occupational field so that the interview can be as realistic as possible. We also urge them to explain the use of the recorder and point out that most employers are impressed when they see someone who is actively pursuing and overcoming a problem.

With clients who are in their early teens we introduce modifications to the standard transfer assignments which are more compatible with their age and interests.

Personalized Transfers

When the clients are about half way through their standard transfers we ask them to develop a list of 10 situations which they feel need particular practice. One client, for instance, might have great difficulty answering the phone and giving his name. He is then encouraged to generate situations wherein other people call his number so that he must answer the telephone and give his name. Another client might have particular difficulty addressing a group meeting in his office. With the clinician's help he could devise a series of graded situations which start in the clinic and gradually approximate conditions in the office. As before, clients are required to record all assignments, analyze their tapes, complete a record form, submit the tapes to the clinician for analysis and discuss their performance with her.

Comments on Transfer

Within the schedule of the intensive clinic we find that clients can work effectively on transfers only 3 to 4 hours per day as it is physically and emotionally exhausting. During the remainder of the day we stabilize correct speech production in the clinic, discuss previous transfer assignments and plan future activities. These in-clinic sessions are also used to review the importance of meeting challenges, the need for careful self-monitoring and the development of positive, constructive attitudes toward transfer activities.

In general, most clients look forward to the transfer phase and move through with little difficulty. This may, of course, be related to the fact that at the end of the establishment phase their speech generally sounds normal in the clinic and their self-confidence is exceedingly high. As they experience success in the early, relatively easy situations, they gain confidence in their ability to handle the job interview at the end.

We've naturally encountered some difficulties in transfer. One problem relates to the mechanics of recording and the production of good quality tapes. Some clients will need extra assistance in this area. A few clients have had such difficulties with entering transfer situations and analyzing their performance that we've assigned a clinician to accompany them in the early situations. In some cases clients have required additional practice in the clinic before they are ready for transfer situations.

We have found that clients usually complete all of the standard transfer assignments within the three week intensive clinic. If they do not have time to finish all the personal assignments we ask them to complete them at home and mail the tapes and record forms to us.

In general, we are very pleased with the transfer program as most clients move through it with minimum difficulties and acquire a firm basis for subsequent maintenance activities.

Maintenance of Fluency Program

The maintenance of a satisfactory level of fluency in the client's post-treatment environment is the final and ultimate target of any treatment program. It is toward this goal that all the rehabilitation strategies are aimed, the raison d'être for all activities.

Maintenance of newly established fluency will not happen automatically. It must be planned carefully and systematic procedures need to be developed. The need for maintenance activities is stressed throughout our clinical program; indeed it is first mentioned in the information package which is sent out to people when they inquire about the program. The importance of long-term maintenance permeates the intensive clinic. Activities in the clinic are arranged to support and illustrate the concept of maintenance.

Our maintenance program consists of a variety of scheduled clinic visits and home programs. The visits include a five-day booster session, evening visits and refresher weekends. Clients are also asked to follow a home program of daily recording, speech assignments and self evaluation. The clinic visits and home program will be described later in this chapter. I will first present a diagramatic representation of a model we have used to help clients conceptualize the need for long term maintenance. This will be followed by statements of principles found to be beneficial in helping clients understand the rationale for maintenance activities. In clinical practice these principles are not presented as discrete entities but are illustrated, demonstrated and supported by a wide variety of activities throughout the treatment program.

In order to help clients appreciate the need for continual self-monitoring and regular practice in the post-treatment environment we have developed the following diagram. The model and accompanying explanation are non-behavioral. The concepts embodied in the explanation are probably untestable but we have observed that it helps clients understand important ideas.

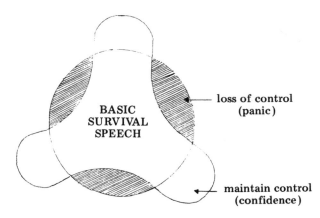

FIGURE 1. Basic Survival Speech

In Figure 1 the circle represents Basic Survival Speech. This refers to that minimum level of fluency that each client needs to cope with speech requirements in his vocational and social environment. It is the level required to hold down a job or engage in elementary social activities such as ordering a restaurant meal. This level will vary for each person. The teacher, lawyer or receptionist will likely need a higher level of fluency to survive a day than will a construction worker or a night watchman.

Although this concept appears vague clients readily attach meaning to it.

The undulating line in Figure 1 represents periodic fluctuations in disfluency. Although the reasons for such fluctuations are unclear, several clinicians have observed that stuttering does occur in waves. In confirmation of this, clients will often report that on their "good" days they can cope with any challenge, they can use all their speech skills correctly, they can vary their rate, and they have little fear of stuttering. They maintain control. On other days, the "bad" days, nothing works. They may as well have stayed in bed. When the line moves **inside** the circle into the shaded areas, this represents those situations or days when the client has trouble, when he cannot speak with sufficient fluency to do his job adequately. It is during these moments/days that the stutterer feels he has lost control and tends toward despair and panic. This is the time when they might feel that all is lost, that they are sliding into the abyss of fear and avoidance which leads back to the vicious cycle of stuttering.

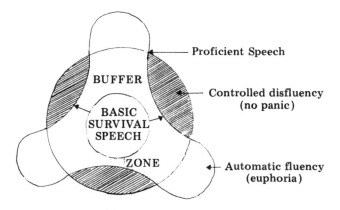

FIGURE 2. Proficient Speech and Buffer Zone

In Figure 2 an outer circle has been added to form a buffer zone. This outer circle represents proficient speech, a level of fluency which is adequate for any situation the client might meet. The client moves from the inner to the outer circle and establishes a buffer zone when his speech reaches the level of proficiency where he can handle situations well beyond those he may meet in his daily routine. An analogy is made to the athlete or professional musician who must exercise or practice daily in order to keep fit. The concert violinist knows that under pressure of public performance he will play less well than when practicing alone in his studio. Therefore, he must attain such a level of excellence in his practice studio that even if he plays less well on the stage, his performance will still satisfy the audience. In the same manner, the client must constantly push himself beyond the minimal requirements so that his performance, under social pressure, will still be satisfactory. He needs to build a buffer zone between what he can do when he really extends himself and what he will need in his daily routine. He must know that even if he experiences disfluencies he is still in control, there is no need to panic. If he knows that he can handle difficult speech situations far beyond what he will likely encounter, this knowledge will give him a secure base of self-confidence and he will believe that he can handle normal requirements as they arise. A maintenance program is a program designed to keep the client in the outer circle with a comfortable buffer zone between himself and panic. The daily routine, exercises and clinic visits are one way for him to keep fit, to live in the outer circle. When the client is functioning in the outer circle of proficient speech, the fluctuations will still occur but now they do not threaten the Basic Survival Speech. Even if he has a "bad" day his speech will still be adequate for his job and social interactions. In this way he will avoid the panic which leads to despair.

In the following section I will outline the principles we develop as we discuss maintenance and prepare clients for the post-clinic period. The points will be presented briefly. Each clinician will need to develop her own style of presenting and illustrating these points.

1. During the final week many clients will display no stuttering in the clinic building and no stuttering or minimal stuttering in outside situations. This degree of fluency will lead some clients to conclude that they are no longer stutterers, that they are cured. In spite of our continued assurances to the contrary they really do believe that stuttering now belongs to the past. The accompanying euphoria is understandable. The unfortunate part, and one that the clinician must guard against, is that the client may conclude that it is no longer necessary for him to monitor and practice his newly acquired

fluency skills.

2. Some degree of relapse will likely occur after the client leaves the clinic. Most people are aware of the way in which particular environmental circumstances control particular behaviors. Stuttering is under strong stimulus control. It is often cued by telephones, speaking in large groups and a host of other situations. In the same manner fluency or controlled speech will come under environmental control. The fluent speech acquired in the clinic will be under the control of the room, the equipment, the building, the clinician and other group members. As long as the client speaks in the presence of all these controlling stimuli he will speak fluently. When a large portion of the environmental stimuli which controlled his speech behavior in the clinic are modified or absent, his speech behavior is likely to be altered. The clinician and client both need to understand this and be prepared for it. There will likely be other changes in his post-clinical environment. The strong support offered by other group members (and the clinician) in the clinic will be gone and replaced by interactions with people who may not be nearly as supportive of the new speech behaviors and who may be less tolerant of the client's attempts at self-monitoring and self-correction. When considering all the changes from the clinical to the post-clinical environment it is not surprising that stutterers sometimes revert to pre-clinical struggle behavior in the post-clinical environment.

3. The level of fluency will fluctuate. There are ample clinical reports that stuttering appears in waves, a period of minimal stuttering will be followed by a period with more difficulty. There is a dearth of research evidence why this happens. It may be related to physiological cycles; or it may be psychological or it may involve some combination thereof. Clients report that during the post-treatment period there will be days when they feel "stuttery," that they anticipate difficulty when just thinking about a situation. It may well be that the cycles are triggered by this anticipation of difficulty with the subsequent struggle and avoidance leading to a self-fulfillment of their predictions.

It may be that stuttering will covary with events in their lives such as job stress, domestic tensions, etc. Clinicians need to caution clients that these cycles are expected, are probably typical and do not indicate failure.

4. Clients need to develop the ability to experience occasional stuttering with subsequent recovery. Due to the pervasive effect of environmental cues for the old stuttering behaviors, the lack of cues for the newly acquired speech, and the nature of habit strength, it is almost inevitable that under conditions of stress, fatigue, excitement, etc., stutterers will revert to previously learned responses of struggle behavior. It is important to help the client focus on the many successes he has and not dwell obsessively on occasional difficulties. If he understands the reasons for reversions to previous struggle behaviors he is more likely to be patient and accept the long term efforts required for maintenance of fluency.

5. The client learns to adapt his speech to different situations. During the last week we teach clients to vary the speech rate from a slow rate of approximately 110 spm to a normal rate of 200 spm. When he expects difficulty in a situation he is advised to adopt the slower rate. The slowed rate provides him a better opportunity to monitor himself and concentrate on employing his newly acquired fluency skills. He returns to the normal speech rate when he feels capable of doing so. We use the analogy of shifting to a lower gear, in a car equipped with a stick shift, when the driver encounters rough terrain. This homely example is readily understood by clients.

6. The client needs to establish realistic targets and communicate these to family and friends. Rather than aiming for 100% fluency in his post-treatment environment we advise clients to set a goal of 97% or 98% fluency. By allowing themselves a reasonable margin of error they remove the pressure for perfection and permit themselves to experiment with error correction as needed. When the client allows himself some room for errors he is more likely to be willing to take the time to monitor himself, cancel errors and analyze the situation.

We also encourage clients to communicate these expectations to people around them. They should tell their friends that they (the stutterers) are likely to stop and correct an error, use a rate change or any number of fluency skills. When their friends understand why the stutterer is doing this, everyone benefits.

Clients should approach friends and family with the attitude that they are very pleased with the progress they have achieved on their speech but that there is still some way to go. Their friends should be notified that from time to time the stutterers will be doing specific things with their speech to maintain fluency. The client may occasionally stutter but with an important difference: before the clinic he was at the mercy of the stutter; now he is in control and will handle the situation more calmly and objectively. Although it is a difficult thing to do, if they can communicate this type of attitude to their friends, they will have gone a long way toward establishing an environment in which they are free to make mistakes, recover from these mistakes and generally profit from errors.

By way of contrast the very worst attitude that clients might adopt is to pretend to their associates that they are now cured, that they no longer stutter. It is easy to understand why stutterers want to adopt this attitude but clinicians must caution against it. If clients adopt the attractive role of a normal speaker, which they might do at the end of an intensive clinic, they will almost certainly generate subsequent difficulties for themselves. If they have assumed the role of a normal speaker and their associates have begun to accept them as such, this will generate almost unbearable pressure to maintain this image. The client will try desperately to keep up this facade of fluency, even to the extent that he will begin to avoid again, use distracting devices and all the familiar tricks of the stutterer. If he has created an environment where he feels under intense pressure to be fluent, he is far less likely to do the things which are so necessary if he is to maintain a satisfactory level of fluency.

I recall an accountant who entered our clinic some years ago as a severe stutterer. Like several others in the intensive clinics he achieved fluency during the second week. During the final 10 days of the clinic he did not stutter once, even in the most difficult transfer situations we could devise for him. His self-confidence was such that he simply did not believe that he could ever stutter again and rejected our suggestions that he should be prepared for occasional stutters. For several months he worked as chief accountant for a school board, talking to hundreds of people without stuttering, presented budgets to the board and thoroughly enjoyed his new status as a fluent speaker. Then the inevitable happened. In the middle of a board meeting he suddenly stuttered. The unexpectedness of it and the reaction of his audience to the disfluency, from one they had come to view as a fluent speaker, was so unpleasant that he panicked. He called me that same afternoon convinced that the world was collapsing around his ears. His discouragement was such that he slid into a serious relapse, dropped out of touch and only emerged two years later when he enrolled for a refresher clinic. He left that clinic with slightly more realistic standards and has maintained better since that time.

7. The client should take the initiative in establishing a supportive, cooperative environment. Clients assume that other people will help and continue to help if they ask them to. We believe that it is often necessary to employ specific strategies to obtain the type of support the client needs. Most people hesitate to intervene in the affairs of others, to nag and point out shortcomings in the behavior of those around them. (There are some notable exceptions to this.) Even if a client asks his friends to correct him when he fails to cancel an error or remind him to adopt a slower rate the friend is unlikely to persist in such admonitions, particularly if the client shows even the slightest irritation when corrected. It is often helpful if the client acknowledges the friend's contribution or finds some way in which to reinforce his friend. The friend must be thanked in some way so that he knows his efforts are appreciated. The clinician may point out several ways of doing this.

One man in our clinic told his young children that he would pay them 25 cents for each time they caught him in an uncorrected error. The children enjoyed the game and they kept their father on his toes.

Terry developed a unique and effective self-control system in which he relied on his friends. After we had described several self-control strategies to him, he developed one based on a punishment model which he called "the pocket of dimes." Terry announced to his associates in the office that he would carry dimes in his left pocket during the day. Whenever a friend noted a failure to cancel an error, Terry promised to shift a dime from his left to his right pocket. At the end of the week he gave the dimes from his right pocket to his secretary with instructions to forward the money to a religious group of which he disapproved. It was particularly odious for him to support that religious group as he was an atheist.

8. The client needs to prepare himself and his family for a gradual shift in role. When a client moves from a moderate/severe stutterer to a normal sounding speaker in three weeks, this dramatic change has many dimensions. The client finds that he now has the facility for normal speech but he may be somewhat bewildered by resultant changes in his social environment. Now that he can speak normally, he feels that he should participate as a normal speaker in society. Where previously he may have waited for his wife to answer the telephone, order a restaurant meal, or remained a silent member in the office coffeebreak group, he now realizes that he must participate more. Such a shift in role introduces many adjustments. He might not possess the necessary social skills to participate effectively in general social chit chat. If he has been a severe stutterer he may simply not have learned these social skills. Much of the group training in the intensive clinic is aimed at improving this area. We include role playing and we practice introductions, asking for a date, etc.

Secondly, the client's associates will also need to make adjustments. Where previously his friends and family knew a person who rarely participated in discussion, who avoided many situations and assumed a passive role, they now find themselves confronted with that same individual who suddenly wants to participate and may even wish to dominate.

The wife may realize that her husband, who had expected her to conduct all domestic business and take the lead in social situations, now wants to run things. This can lead to many adjustment problems for both husband and wife. One woman stuttered so severely that she resorted to writing notes during the first clinical interview. After the three week clinic her husband returned to find a woman who, excited by her new speech fluency, talked incessantly and became involved in all manner of new activities. It was a difficult adjustment period for both of them. We referred them to a marriage counselor who helped them through this period.

The clinician needs to alert clients to potential difficulties in these areas, provide whatever direction and counseling she can to the families and refer to other agencies as needed.

9. The client must take positive action toward changing his life style. If they wish to cultivate and develop a new image of

themselves as persons who participate actively in verbal situations, they need to move into environments which permit and support the development of those skills. They are encouraged to join clubs, discussion groups and public speaking courses. We urge them to seek a promotion within their field of work or move into a vocation with more opportunities to use their new speech skills. An additional benefit of such changes is that they will form new social circles where expectations are likely to be more in line with their current self-concept, of a person who participates in verbal interactions, who may occasionally experience some speech difficulties but can handle them. The more successful they are in establishing themselves with new friends, new and expanded job responsibilities, the less likely they are to return to the old role of withdrawal and isolation. This is not meant to imply that they should abandon their former friends but rather that they should adopt a goal of expansion and enrichment throughout their life.

Home Maintenance Program

When we present the home program we reiterate that it is necessary to develop a regular practice schedule in order to keep fit and maintain a buffer zone. Although the home assignments are fairly specific, we suggest that these assignments be viewed as guidelines and that each client should develop a home program to suit his particular needs. We also assume that clients will vary in their willingness and capacity to carry out home programs. We have, therefore, developed three home programs. Plan A requires approximately one hour each day; Plan B about 40 minutes; Plan C about 20 minutes. Each client should determine how much time he is able and willing to spend and then make every effort to fulfill that commitment. If a client has limited time available it is far better that he select a short program which he can complete than a longer program which he cannot complete. The clinician may need to help clients develop a realistic home program.

To implement the home program the client will need a tape recorder. We also ask clients to purchase a wrist counter which is capable of recording instances of behavior. After each assignment has been completed, clients analyze the tape and record the activity on the maintenance record form.

Plan A—Daily Speech Activities:

1. Every morning and evening you should read or speak for two minutes at approximately 100 syllables/min. and for two minutes at 200 syllables/min. Record the speech, listen to the playback with special attention to the smoothness of your speech. If you detect any tension or struggle you should repeat the exercise. You should strive to sound **and** feel like a normal speaker.

2. Start the first two conversations of each day at approximately 120 spm and then gradually increase to the normal rate.

3. Keep a careful record of the total number of stutters each day. Record them on your wrist counter and then transfer the total to the tables and graphs at the end of each day. This activity will be difficult to maintain so you will need to develop an effective system of self reward for your efforts. The rationale for this is that it permits you to observe trends in your speech across time.

4. Engage in a five-minute conversation with a family member or friend. Record the conversation, analyze it and record the total number of stutterings. Remember to cancel errors.

5. Do five personal assignments each day and record the results. These assignments should be structured around situations you find most difficult.

All of the assignments will take approximately one hour each day to complete and record. You will need to develop a daily schedule which allows for this each day. Excuses are easy to make but will have sad consequences.

After we have described Plan A to the clients we urge them to consider committing the necessary time at home. If they predict that they will be unable to spend the necessary time for Plan A we introduce Plan B and Plan C.

Each of these plans has progressively fewer activities and requires less time to complete. Whatever plan they choose they are urged to stick to it. We also provide record forms for them to complete at home and urge them to make entries on a regular basis.

Booster Sessions

Two years ago we introduced a five-day booster session on a trial basis. This session was scheduled at the end of the summer and would thus occur one to three months after clients had completed the intensive clinics scheduled from May through July. We invite everyone to attend the booster session in the same summer as they take the intensive clinic. Sometimes clients are not able to do this so they may attend in a subsequent year. During the booster session clients obtain additional practice on the various fluency skills introduced during the establishment phase. The main emphasis, however, is upon self-monitoring and analysis, self-management skills and the maintenance principles as outlined above.

Evening Visits and Refresher Weekends

Immediately after the intensive clinic clients return for weekly evening visits. After four weeks these are re-scheduled to monthly meetings and then stopped after four months. We also schedule refresher weekends at one month intervals throughout the year. The weekends are open to any clients who have completed the intensive courses in previous years. They begin Saturday morning and continue until Sunday afternoon. The weekends are essentially telescoped versions of the intensive clinics with practice in prolonged speech rates, rate changes, fluency skills, self-analysis and transfer assignments. Clients also participate in debates, discuss their experiences in the post-treatment environment and work toward improving their self-management skills.

We also use the refresher weekends as an opportunity to evaluate the clients' post-clinic speech. At the beginning of the weekend session each client is recorded as he makes several phone calls to strangers. These tapes are then analyzed and converted to syllable rate and percentage of stuttering. We have also started to make "surprise" phone calls to clients in their homes or at their work. These phone calls are recorded and analyzed. We have observed that there is usually some difference between the speech of a client when he returns to the clinic and when he answers an unexpected phone call at work or in his home.

Comments on Maintenance

Maintenance programs are difficult to conduct, require a great deal of patience and can sometimes be downright discouraging. There are numerous problems which we have not yet solved. There is the problem of what we should measure to determine our success. Even if we knew what to measure we would still need to know how to measure it, when to measure it and where. Another set of problems revolves around logistic considerations. Clients are scattered around a very large country and have diverse and busy schedules. Moreover, it is often difficult to find clinical staff for evening and weekend work which seems to be necessary in a maintenance program.

In addition to the practical problems alluded to above there are several theoretical issues which remain unsolved. Should we concentrate on teaching self-control and self-management skills so that clients can arrange their own environment more effectively? Or, should we work toward over-training and over-learning in the clinic so that the newly acquired responses will be resistant to extinction in the post-clinic environment? Or, should we strive to increase the effectiveness that the support clients might derive from family and friends; in effect, produce lay therapists in the client's home environment?

Each of these three approaches, and there may be several more, is theoretically feasible but we need massive amounts of clinical research to tell us which way to direct our efforts. Perhaps a combination of all three approaches will provide the most effective approach.

In spite of the problems outlined above I am heartened by the progress that the profession has realized in the last few years. Most people now recognize that maintenance is not automatic, that it must be planned for. Many people have started serious and systematic investigations of several dimensions in maintenance. I am optimistic that these trends will continue and expand as professionals come to view maintenance as the most important phase of the rehabilitation of stutterers. Within our own clinic I'm also encouraged. More and more clients return after several years of fluctuations to report that they are beginning to understand what they must do if they want to maintain a satisfactory level of fluency. Although many clients report rough times of despair and discouragement we hear more and more clients say that they now know that they will survive and continue to make progress toward a satisfactory level of fluency.

References

Boberg, E., Howie, P., and Woods, L., "Maintenance of Fluency: A Review" in *Journal of Fluency Disorders*, 4, 93-116, 1979.

Boberg, E. (Ed.), *Maintenance of Fluency*. New York: Elsevier North-Holland, Inc., 1981.

Boberg, E. and Kully, D., "Techniques for Transferring Fluency" in Perkins (Ed.), *Current Therapy of Communication Disorders*. New York: Thieme-Stratton, In Press.

Boberg, E. and Kully, D., *Comprehensive Alberta Stuttering Program*. In Press.

Goldberg, S., *Behavioral Cognitive Stuttering Therapy*. Tigard, Oregon: C. C. Publications, 1981.

Howie, P., Tanner, S., and Andrews, G., "Short and Long-term Outcome in an Intensive Treatment Program for Adult Stutterers," in *Journal of Speech and Hearing Disorders*, 46, 104-109, 1981.

Ingham, R., and Andrews, G., "Details of a Token Economy Stuttering Therapy Program for Adults" in *Australian Journal of Human Communication Disorders*, 1, 13-20, 1973.

Ingham, R., "The Effects of Self-Evaluation Training on Maintenance and Generalization During Stuttering Treatment" in *Journal of Speech and Hearing Disorders*, 47, 271-280, 1982.

Perkins, W. H., "Replacement of Stuttering with Normal Speech: I. Rationale," in *Journal of Speech and Hearing Disorders*, 38, 283-294, 1973.

Perkins, W. H., "Replacement of Stuttering with Normal Speech: II. Clinical Procedures" in *Journal of Speech and Hearing Disorders*, 38, 295-303, 1973.

Perkins, W. H. (Ed.), "Strategies in Stuttering Therapy, Volume 1, No. 4 in *Seminars in Speech, Language and Hearing*, 1980.

Ryan, B, in Thomas, Charles C. (Ed.), *Programmed Therapy for Stuttering in Children and Adults*. Springfield, IL: 1974.

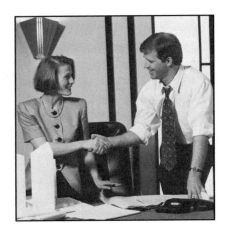

chapter four

An Alternative to Automatic Fluency

by William H. Perkins, Ph.D.

The roads to recovery from stuttering are varied. Some recover "spontaneously" for reasons not fully understood. Some recover with the help of therapy, especially if they are young children. Some only improve temporarily. For those whose fluency does not become automatic and expressively spontaneous, "controlled" fluency is an alternative. The questions of automaticity of fluent speech, of whether automaticity can be achieved through therapy, and of maintenance of "controlled" fluency with its requirement of monitoring are the topics of this chapter.

Automatic Fluency

For many, perhaps most, who stutter, the dream is freedom from stuttering, freedom from fear of stuttering, and freedom from even having to think about stuttering and fluency. For those who recover spontaneously, apparently the vast majority, this freedom becomes a fact. One way or another, they "outgrow" their stuttering, usually before puberty but sometimes during adolescence. Typically, they no longer think of themselves as stutterers. Similar outcomes are also reported for children who stutter who have recovered with the help of therapy. Even some whose stuttering has persisted into adulthood have, with the help of a variety of therapies ranging from psychotherapies to behavior therapies, gained sufficient fluency that their speech is not considered a problem.

For people in all of these groups, stuttering would appear to be cured. They no longer think of themselves as stutterers. They have not lost control of their speech for such a long time that when they are disfluent, their hesitancies and repetitions are experienced as normal gropings for words and phrases. The expectation of becoming involuntarily blocked has become such a distant memory that it has long since ceased to be paralyzing. Stuttering does not play a major, or even minor, role in their lives. Fluency and normal disfluency have become so automatic that they think of their speech as being normal and of themselves as being normal speakers.

The fact that such complete recovery can occur, even in some cases in people who stuttered severely, raises the baffling question of how it was possible. They show no signs of having to use control techniques to preserve fluency or to prevent stuttering. Is a change of attitude and self-image all that is needed? Perhaps. Certainly, this possibility can not be excluded. What is apparently excluded, at least for these people, is a defective motor speech mechanism which requires continuous use of compensatory techniques to preserve normal fluency.

There is another road to automatic fluency, however, that is treacherous for many. In the early years of our use of rate control to shape fluency, we observed a form of normal speech that we came to call "lucky fluency." It routinely occurred after rate was accelerated from the slow drone, with which shaping began, to a fast fluent drone, the only form of controlled speech that was then available with rate procedures. To accelerate beyond the rate limits of a fast drone, rate controls had to be relinquished.

Invariably, what followed was a period of normal fluency. It was, of course, the type of fluency these people had dreamed of: it required no controls, no attention; it was as if by magic they could speak fluently. It lasted typically for a few days, sometimes only hours, sometimes weeks, and in one case for over two years. When relapse occurred, as it eventually did, the disappearance of lucky fluency was as magical as its appearance. Because these people did nothing over which they had control to produce their automatic fluency, they had no tools for recovering it when it vanished.

Needless to say, we became suspicious of it as a treatment outcome to be encouraged. Still, it occurred so regularly that we had to contend with the probability that it would happen sooner or later. Admittedly, it was attractive while it lasted. It not only sounded like normal speech, it also felt like normal speech because it did not require attention and control of fluency to achieve. We decided it was better discovered during, rather than after, treatment. At least that gave us a chance to reestablish fluency with skills that were under voluntary control. The resulting speech sounded reasonably normal, but it was far from automatic.

What can be learned from lucky fluency? Probably not much for certain, other than the fact that it is not a reliable basis for achieving long term freedom from stuttering. The questions it generates are better than any answers it provides. For example, why does it occur in the first place? Is it because the motor feeling of stutter-free speech established with fluency skills is strong enough to launch a period of automatic fluency, however brief? Perhaps. Or is it because of confidence in being able to speak fluently? Perhaps.

Even of more interest is the question of why lucky fluency ends. Is it because confidence in being able to speak normally is eroded to the point of relapse? Perhaps. Could automatic fluency be preserved if the person has confidence that, with easily used fluency skills, normal-sounding speech is assured whenever automatic fluency fails? Perhaps.

This possibility, that fluency skills assure normal-sounding speech, was not really tested when our only fluency skill was rate control. With it, the resultant drone was often less desirable than stuttering. The only answer that seems reasonably clear from our experience with lucky fluency agrees with the conclusion we reached earlier about recovered stutterers. It is that relapse can probably not be blamed on a defective motor speech mechanism. While lucky fluency prevails, speech is automatically fluent, normally expressive, and speech rates are at least normally, and sometimes excessively, fast. This is not the picture one would expect to see, even on a temporary basis, if techniques were being used to compensate for impaired motor speech equipment.

Achieving Automatic Fluency

Can a bridge be built from controlled normal-sounding speech to automatic fluency? The answer is necessarily speculative. If the motor speech mechanism is impaired in ways that preclude fluency at normal rates and with normal expressiveness, as seems to be the case in some instances of brain injury, then the answer is probably "no." Automatically expressive speech seems to be biologically mandated so near the upper limits of maximum rate that speeds slow enough to preserve fluency probably have to be monitored consciously. On the other hand, we have just argued that people who have recovered from stuttering spontaneously, or who have enjoyed periods of lucky fluency, show no signs of being unable to speak rapidly and expressively. Whatever the causes of their stuttering, they appear to be capable of automatic fluency.

Apparently, then, some who stutter, perhaps most, have the potential for recovery. How can it be accomplished? Not only is that the question we are addressing here, it has been addressed in conferences, texts, and clinical research. It is the thorniest of clinical problems in its resistance to effective solutions.

For fluency-skill programs, at least, the cost/effectiveness ratio seems to be the biggest hurdle to permanence. On the cost side, the vigilance required to maintain fluency becomes tiresome. Vacations from vigilance are tempting, and with each vacation, stuttering is likely to recur. On the effectiveness side, any weakening of the motivation for fluency is an invitation to a vacation from vigilance. Thus, any tilting of the ratio to the cost side works against maintenance of fluency.

Achieving automatic fluency would appear to be an instance of the general issue of automatization of a motor skill. A large body of theory and research has grown around this issue. Motor schema theory, for example, emphasizes the necessity of stabilizing an image of the desired skill over and above the movements involved in the skill. Neurologically, evidence exists that the number of neurons needed to perform an act voluntarily is significantly reduced when that act becomes automatic.

As far as replacing stuttering with fluency is concerned, the motor speech problem is how to replace an automatic response rehearsed for most of a lifetime, with a voluntary response that requires almost constant attention to maintain. That this could require as long as five years of diligent practice is suggested by a laryngectomee who was determined to sound like a normal speaker. He practiced various inflections of a phrase 1,000 times a day, every day, for five years before the quality of esophageal speech he sought became automatic.

One could argue that it took him so long because he had to learn such drastically different skills. One could also argue that the stutterer faces a tougher task because, with no effort, he can lapse back to stuttering, whereas the laryngectomee has only one option, esophageal speech, to rehearse. Although recurrence of an old automatic response like stuttering may not retard automatization of fluency, it certainly does not hasten the process.

In all likelihood, more is required than motor-speech skills in the replacement of stuttering with automatic fluency. Clearly, chronic stuttering involves a set of expectations about speech, and probably about life in general, that are virtually an integral part of the stuttering. Availability of controlled fluency after a brief period of therapy, often very brief, cannot be expected to alter a life style forged across many years. One is likely to remain on guard, with the old apprehensions and avoidance tactics in reserve, as long as the secret conviction is held that stuttering is still waiting to strike at unexpected moments.

Presumably, what is needed to alter this conviction is a period in which speech free of stuttering is maintained with skills low enough in cost to make the price of fluency acceptable. The assumption is that with an acceptable alternative to stuttering, fear of its occurrence will diminish and eventually become extinct. With confidence that speech is manageable, including the new conviction that even disfluencies resembling the old stuttering blockages will not spiral out of control, the achievement of automatic fluency is at hand.

Therapy Requirements for Automatic Fluency.   A four

part therapy program is probably needed to facilitate reaching the goal of automatic fluency. This would include a skill program that effectively provides fluency with low cost in monitoring and control of speech; a transfer and maintenance program that maximizes motivation for preservation of fluency; a counseling program that is aimed at disproving the conviction that speech is treacherously difficult, and that helps to adjust the self-image accordingly; and for some, a program in speaking skills that will provide experience in mastering the subtleties of conversational give and take among fluent speakers.

A low-cost fluency skill program needs to provide normal-sounding speech with relatively little attention to use of the skill needed to preserve that speech. Each of the options has its advantages and disadvantages. Syllable prolongation, for example, is the most universally effective technique for establishing fluency, but the price is a drone. To achieve normal-sounding speech with this fluency skill requires training in normally expressive rhythms of speech stress. Thus, it is a relatively high-cost skill with which to preserve fluency.

Breath management skills, on the other hand, do not necessarily distort speech rate or expressiveness very much, and they are relatively easy to use. With males, however, who are concerned with having a masculine-sounding voice, the social consequences of a breathy voice can be severe. Moreover, some who stutter, especially if they stutter severely, are not able to establish fluency with breath skills alone.

A transfer and maintenance program needs to provide an efficient system for extending fluency, maintained by fluency skills, from the clinic to successful use in daily life. An operant self-management program has been reported with which fluency has been successfully maintained. It involves training in self-evaluation of fluency. Progress to increased spacing of maintenance sessions depends on successful preservation of fluency.

A counseling program is needed to help stutterers search out their secret avoidances with which they preserve the conviction that their speech will become involuntarily blocked if they are not constantly vigilant. This will probably require discovering that they can cope with stresses that have triggered stuttering in the past without fear that such disfluencies as do occur will escalate into involuntary blockages.

A speaking skills program is needed for those whose stuttering has interfered with developing facility in the give and take of conversational life. These are subtle skills that depend on timing and techniques for entering and sustaining conversational exchanges. Establishment of fluency does not automatically alter one's tactics for managing conversational exchanges that may have developed around a lifetime of severe stuttering.

An Alternative to Automatic Fluency

In our experience, automatic fluency does not typically result from use of fluency skills. Perhaps those skills have not been used long enough or diligently enough for fluency to become habitual. Perhaps the skills used have exacted too high a price in the amount of attention required to maintain fluency. Perhaps the conviction that stuttering is a permanent part of their lives has been so strong that it has resisted extinction by the availability of fluency. Or perhaps the motivation for fluency has weakened.

Whatever the reason, we observed year after year that the most predictable results of therapy were like this. First, a temporary period of lucky fluency occurred soon after slow normal speech was achieved. This period was followed by vigorous work on fluency skills as recognition grew that lucky fluency left them vulnerable to relapse without the necessary skills for recovery. After fluency was transferred to daily life, many were all but ecstatic with their speech. A year or more later, most were pleased, but few were still thrilled. Some used their skills frequently, but none used them constantly. The overall long-term result was that 75 percent considered their speech to be improved, but only a few no longer had to worry about stuttering.

We eventually concluded that we had two alternatives in our maintenance activities. One was to help develop more powerful motivation for preservation of fluency. We decided against this alternative because it puts us in the position of extolling the merits of fluency. We decided that these merits were doubtless already evident to those who presumably had more at stake in recognizing them than we did. Recognizing that the option of replacing stuttering with normal-sounding controlled speech might not be as attractive year in and year out as it seemed to us, we decided in favor of freedom-of-choice rather than exhortation. With this decision, our goal of therapy shifted away from attempts to preserve fluency in those who clearly did not choose to use their fluency skills diligently enough to remain stutter-free.

What our goal of therapy for these people became was to demonstrate to them that, with use of fluency skills, they could sound like normal speakers in any condition in which they expected to stutter. **Thus, our goal of maintenance is not to preserve fluency; rather, it is to preserve fluency skills with which normal-sounding speech is available whenever needed or wanted.** With these skills intact, fluency is a realistic option to stuttering in any situation. Freedom-of-choice is upheld.

Because continual use of fluency throughout therapy implies that our expectation is permanent continuation of that fluency, a modification was needed in our transfer procedures. What is now included in those procedures is practice in discontinuation of fluency-skill use until stuttering occurs, and then practice in recovery of fluency. Naturally, the reason for this procedure, which on the face of it seems contradictory to the purpose of therapy, requires explanation.

Protestations of commitment to fluency for life are often voiced at this point. Our response is not to discourage pursuit of the option of permanent fluency. Instead, we indicate that this recovery procedure is intended to strengthen the conviction of these people that they can remain in control of their speech under all circumstances.

We say, in effect, "If you know from experience that you can recover from a recurrence of stuttering, then you are less likely to fear a complete relapse." On the other hand, we say, "If you leave our clinic with experience only in being fluent, then you have no certainty that you would be able to recover were speech to break down." (We do not emphasize the probability of this breakdown.) "This uncertainty will likely be a nagging fear that we want you to prove to yourself is unnecessary. You can do this by permitting yourself to stutter in the toughest situations you can find, and then, by using your fluency skills, demonstrate your ability to recover normal-sounding speech."

By the time these people are ready for recovery practice,

they will have mastered several fluency skills, including syllable-prolongation, shortened phrase length, easy voice onset, breathy voice, articulatory blending of one sound into the next, and normally expressive rhythmic patterns. They also may have worked on relaxed breathing, and kinesthetic awareness of tension as anticipation of stuttering approaches.

Although they will have used all of these techniques in conjunction with each other to insure establishment of fluency at slow rates, they will select only one or two of them that work best at normally rapid rates. Obviously, to control speech by using all of these skills simultaneously would be a gross exercise in overkill. It would be to invite paralysis by analysis. With the emphasis on maintenance of skills rather than on maintenance of fluency, all of the skills are practiced so that they remain available when, and if, needed.

A merit of this alternative to the goal of automatic fluency is that it does not preclude approaching that goal. In fact, it facilitates the approach. Pressure is reduced on the necessity of preserving fluency, and fear of stuttering is reduced by successful use of fluency skills to recover from it. Rather than a frontal assault, this is a flanking maneuver in which progressively extended periods of fluency occur as the result of successful recoveries from stuttering. Arrival at automatic fluency is more by accident than intent.

The objective is to be able to sound normally fluent when needed, and for many, this may be as far as they go. But for some, ability to recover from stuttering may be so successful that fear of becoming involuntarily blocked dwindles to insignificance. For them, the day may come when they discover by surprise that they are not only free from stuttering, they are also free from fear of stuttering, and free from even having to think much about speech.

A Postscript on Measuring Progress

What you measure is not necessarily what you get. Progress is routinely recorded with objective measures, especially in these days of accountability. A variety of objective measures are used ranging from frequency of words stuttered, to frequency of broken words, to frequency of sound repetitions, prolongations, and hesitations. Important as these measures are, they often do not tell the whole story, or even an important part of it.

A few years ago, we sent over 150 questionnaires to people who had graduated from our program one to five years earlier. We wanted honest answers to questions about the effects of therapy on their lives as well as on their speech. Accordingly, we asked that their questionnaires be anonymous. Karl's was typical of the first five that were returned. We were ready to close the clinic after reading them. Karl, for example, was dissatisfied with his speech when he graduated, and was now very dissatisfied. He obviously wanted us to know who he was, because his name was emblazoned above his responses. Having his name, we checked our records for his performance. Before therapy, his speech was distinctly blocked when he stuttered, but this only occurred on about 12 percent of his syllables. After therapy, disfluencies were reduced to 2 percent, and none involved blockage. By objective standards, Karl was a success. Although the vast majority of the responses received were congruent with our objective measures, the need was driven home to us, by Karl and a few others, to evaluate how the people we have seen feel about the help we have tried to provide, as well as how they have actually performed.

The other reservation about measurement to be noted here is that stuttering may get lost in the record keeping. A number of problems exist. For example, many laymen make a distinction between stuttering and stammering, but for decades speech pathologists have lumped them together under "stuttering." That is how they identify the problem when they ask for a judgment.

We found out, to our chagrin, that this usage can be confusing. At least it was to the school teachers whom we asked to identify forms of disfluency that they considered to be stuttering. The results were puzzling until we discovered, by accident, that many of these teachers thought that we wanted them just to identify stuttering, not stammering. Accordingly, the most severe blockages were not identified as stuttering because our judges considered them to be stammering. Admittedly, this is more of a problem in research than in clinical practice, but it is associated with the larger issue of whether any of our methods of measuring stuttering are valid.

For clinical purposes, as well as for research, stuttering has been considered to be what observers can agree among themselves to call stuttering. A curious consequence of this method of defining stuttering is that the speaker is not privileged to render his judgment about his own moment of stuttering when it occurs. That experience is his, so no one else can verify it. He can participate in judging afterward by listening to a recording of his performance; this judgment can be verified. What is excluded, then, from any acceptable definition of stuttering is whether or not a speech interruption reflects linguistic uncertainty or loss of speech control.

Some of us have been so concerned about reliably identifying stuttering that we have tried to improve it by removing as much ambiguity from the judgment as possible. What we have done is to arbitrarily take any form of syllable disfluency as an operational measure of stuttering. The effect of this strategy can sometimes be weird. We have, for instance, occasionally worked with people who had only one or two severe blocks during an initial interview. The remainder of their speech was completely fluent. After therapy, when they felt that their speech was free of stuttering, it then included normal disfluency. The change in objective performance by which we recorded this progress showed less than 1 percent syllable disfluency before treatment and more than 2 percent at termination. By "objective" standards, stuttering would appear to have increased as a result of therapy.

This is not intended as an argument against the need for reliable measures of speech performance. We continue to use the best measures available. What concerns us is that we may be sacrificing valid identification of stuttering for reliable judgments. As clinicians, we try to remain alert to the possibility that the true experience of stuttering may only be known by the speaker, not by the listener.

References

Ingham, R., "Effects of Self-evaluation Training on Maintenance and Generalization During Stuttering Treatment," *Journal of Speech and Hearing Disorders,* 47, 271—280, 1982.

Kent, R. and Lybolt, J., "Techniques of Therapy Based on Motor Learning Theory," in W. Perkins (Ed.) *Current Therapy of Communication Disorders: General Principles of Therapy.* New York: Thieme-Stratton, Inc., 1982.

Perkins, W., "Replacement of Stuttering with Normal Speech: I. Rationale," *Journal of Speech and Hearing Disorders,* 38, 283—294 (a), 1973.

Perkins, W., "Replacement of Stuttering with Normal Speech: II. Clinical Procedures, *Journal of Speech and Hearing Disorders,* 38, 295—303 (b), 1973.

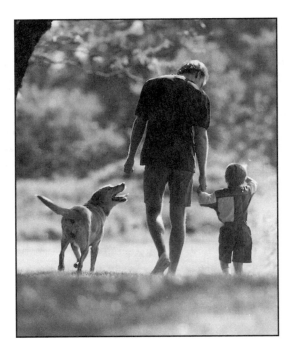

chapter five

Body Concept, Self Concept and Balance

by Elisabeth Versteegh-Vermeij

As a European clinician my background and training differ from those of my American colleagues. Nevertheless we know of major developments in the United States and tend to follow them closely in the Netherlands. What is specifically ours to contribute touches an aspect that I myself deem vital and so I shall try in this chapter to get information back across the ocean. I shall do so by describing the development of our ideas through experience and critical observation. Unfortunately much of the literature on this subject is inaccessible because of the language barrier.[1] As transfer and maintenance are the goals of any therapy, it must be understood that I am keeping them unwaveringly in sight in the following pages, even if it should not appear to be so.

For many years I have worked with stutterers of all ages,

---

[1] I must caution the reader that skill in any kind of therapy can only be acquired by personal practice. This is especially true of body oriented therapy.

both in group therapy and in individual therapy. I have learned from my successes, but not much, since success tends to confirm what one already thinks to be true. However, I have learned enormously from failures; from the observations and experiences that did not fit with my theoretical assumptions; from attitudes and behaviors of stutterers that seemed baffling until I had the courage to see more than meets the eye and hear more than the spoken message. I shall describe in the following pages a dimension to be added to existing, well-developed therapies, from which stutterers already benefit. I have found that this added dimension can make the foundation for transfer and maintenance more solid, thus augmenting the number of stutterers who will profit "for life."

Lack of motivation will be greatly reduced when the stutterer is treated as an indivisible entity. The word "individual" means just that. **This is to say that his body and what it expresses, or fails to express, should be treated with the same care and attention as his mental attitudes or his actual speech behavior. The whole person is both a mind and a body, a unified "system."**

Slowly but inexorably I have come to the conviction that human behavior is much more complex than is suggested by the literature on operant conditioning. Simultaneous processes in mind and body are served by interdependent feedback loops and an energy block in any part of the system influences all other parts. In recent times, many therapies have been developed to reintegrate body and mind, and I am convinced that stuttering therapy also will greatly benefit from this progress.

What works for whom and why? What makes change possible in the first place? What is it that makes new attitudes and behaviors permanent? Is there a common denominator to be found in those who can transfer what they learn in therapy to the complexities of everyday life, or in those who relapse again and again, or in those who do not even begin to change? Which therapy should one choose for which stutterer? As widely differing theoretical approaches seemed to have the same rate of success in practical reality I came to suspect dimly that it is not so much what speech therapy brings to the stutterer as what the stutterer brings to speech therapy that determines the outcome. Over the years this dim suspicion has become a bright conviction.

Body Oriented Therapy

In 1968 I heard of a young couple of speech therapists, Theo and Toni Schoenaker, who had introduced residential group therapy for stuttering in the town of Doetinchem in the Netherlands some years earlier. They introduced not only residential group therapy which met with much opposition at that time but also sensory awareness or "getting in touch with the reality of one's own body." Anatomically well founded and carefully developed "awareness exercises" were used to restore the natural balance between tension and relaxation in posture, movements, and breathing. This concept met with even more opposition than group therapy but as more and more speech clinicians grew convinced of the inherent logic of "bodywork," the concept spread. It has proved to be such a valuable asset and so generally useful, for voice rehabilitation no less than for stuttering therapy, that sensory awareness and elements of bioenergetics are now part of the curriculum in colleges for speech clinicians in the Netherlands.

Their stuttering therapy consists of five stages, each lasting five days, spread out over 6 months with gradually increasing intervals between sessions. There are two therapists and 14-16 clients in each group. Groups of adult stutterers usually consist of people between 20 and 35 years of age with the usual predominance of men. We have groups of teenagers (boys from 12-15 and boys from 15-18) in which parental involvement is stimulated and encouraged. The same is true for the groups of teenage girls. As there are fewer girls who stutter and as girls seem less willing to leave home, it is seldom possible to separate the age groups, but with two clinicians it is possible to work on different levels when that is called for. In the adult groups we have also had men and women in their forties and fifties, who were in no way more difficult to help than the younger ones. Age does not seem to be the prime variable: there have been older people who did not profit just as there have been young people who were too afraid to change.

Stage One

During the first stage of therapy, clients learn to stand

straight and "grounded."[1] They are encouraged not to "take a breath" but to let inhalation just happen and to concentrate rather on **exhaling** fully and easily. The breathing exercises are not meant to facilitate speech as such, but to affirm a person's strength. Becoming aware of tension in feet, legs, back, and neck and experiencing the release of superfluous tensing in favor of resilience take up a major part of the time. Resilience is also the goal of those who are not too tense but who suffer from a lack of healthy tension, who are slumped instead of rigid. Both rigidity and excessive pliability are ways to avoid "being there." Making the client feel his actual strength; making him realize he has a backbone and can stand squarely on his own two feet; letting him experience the easy diaphragmatic breathing which is a natural result of this resilient stance is a major contribution to the buffer zone that another author in this volume has described.

The only way we work on speech as such during this first stage is to let the clients practice stuttering with their eyes open, standing grounded with head held high. For some eye contact is still too difficult, for many it is part of this stage's achievement, at least in the safety of the therapeutic setting. The assignment given to the clients when they leave treatment is to utilize moments of waiting, of walking from one place to another or other opportunities during the day, to **consciously feel the way they stand and move and breathe,** and to do this in an **accepting, friendly, attentive** way. Even changing a slumped posture to a straighter one, or giving up a rigid stance for one of more realistic pliability involves a risk. Any change does. So it is all-important to have the client actively work on feeling strong and courageous. The breathing exercises, which stress **exhalation** are linked to movements of the legs and lower back, to counteract high-thoracical respiration. When this latter pattern of respiration is habitual, it is itself a source of tension. Stamping the feet, and kicking in all directions, are accompanied by phonating with a loud resonant voice; this makes the client feel literally "alive and kicking." Striding towards a group of other stutterers, stopping to ground oneself and then looking at the group, saying

---

[1]The quality of being "grounded" refers to a person's ability to be aware of his own body, an awareness that reaches from the head to the feet in such a way that he even touches the ground more solidly.

in a loud voice: "This is where I stand . . . Here I am . . . My name is . . ." makes the client experience his presence in the here and now with less fear. This is rewarding in itself.

If a person cannot stamp his own foot ("put his foot down") without ever so slightly shaking his head, or frowning or closing his eyes, or in other ways negating what the stamping is meant to express, the clinician must take time for extra encouragement and support and for more training on this level. In each therapy session we keep coming back to this concept of strength and courage, which makes one capable of choosing for oneself instead of giving responsibility for oneself to others. In this context I want to remark that assertiveness training is of restricted value when basic strength is lacking. It is learned as a trick, as a way to manipulate others, and will not be convincing. People find it "doesn't work" for them and indeed it cannot if they have no foundation for the assertiveness to rest on.

Stage Two

The second therapy stage is devoted to another level — that of feeling safe. It is the counterpart, not the opposite, of feeling strong: it is the ability to let go, to trust completely, to intimately accept others into one's life. Rocking, rolling, swaying (as if being moved by wind or water) and very quiet relaxed breathing deep down in the pelvis, enhance feelings of security and the ability to "open up"; either to give or to receive. Relaxing the pelvic area has its counterpart in the relaxation of throat and jaw musculature just as resilience in posture has its counterpart in presence of mind.

In the group, learning to entrust oneself to others and learning to accept others as they trust you is stimulated by working in two's and three's. In many nonverbal training procedures "being together without losing oneself" or "accepting others without holding back" may be experienced. Clients are encouraged to experiment with nonsense syllables ("baby-talk") with loose jaw movements and a minimum of breath. The reader may see the connection between the bodywork of feeling safe enough to let breathing just happen, as natural ebb and flow, and the resulting release of tension in the speech musculature. The assignments for the interval until the next therapy session include taking time for breathing exercises which are devised to loosen the pelvic area, practicing stuttering in easy situations while becoming aware of the body (feeling grounded) and continuing to experiment with the simple, childish attitude in speech. Sheehan's concept of the Iceberg will have been discussed and clients realize at least intellectually how they let themselves be influenced by the standards (real or imagined) of the environment. Depending on how strong or secure they already feel they can start on the road to change. Before leaving they will have experimented with the loose way of talking in relatively simple outside situations. At home they are again expected to make notes and to report on experiences. When these reports are unsatisfactory the conclusion must be drawn that the client is not strong and/or not secure enough to risk changing and more work has to be done to fortify and encourage him. As a therapist I want to respect his defenses. If he still needs them, it is no use forcing him to pretend that he has given them up.

Stage Three

In the next stage we explore emotional blocking. The adult stutterer admits to fear of stuttering. The fact that he "uses" the stuttering not to have to express anger, painful grief, or joy which may make him vulnerable is something he will have great difficulty accepting. He seems out of touch with his feelings when he stutters. The bodywork that has been done before will prove helpful in facing what he has grown too afraid to acknowledge. He needs courage, and a sense of personal worth to risk the confrontation with what has been too dangerous to even consider.

Teaching people who stutter to confront their emotions and to handle them adequately again adds to the buffer zone which makes transfer and maintenance of new speech behaviors possible. When one considers stuttering as in essence the holding back of expressive speech, one can see how important it is to explore the emotional level. Emotions can be mimed and it will be discovered that some clients can express fear but not anger, some can express grief but not joy, and so on. Some are very good mimics because they are good at "role playing," but others cannot express themselves at all because they cannot even **play** at being free. Expressing emotion in nonsense syllables first, then in words in a fictitious situation, then in words that apply to one's own personal difficulties is the progression followed. Clients are advised when experiencing an emotion to breathe deeply and so strengthen the emotion, using the energy this gives to express what one wants to express.

At this point the personal stuttering pattern is analyzed. Clients are asked to leave out one aspect, then another, to imitate each other's stuttering and to feel the difference in what they do themselves. We have found it helpful to imitate the client's stuttering in every detail. Why does one stutter in one's own particular way? What does this stuttering express? What emotional value does it have for the client himself? What made it develop in the way it has? What makes him stick to it? These are the questions asked.

We then come to "easy stuttering" which for us means making the **voice** go towards the listener in a fluent way although the words as such may still be broken. We use easy voice onset, easy repetitions of consonants, not using the "schwa" sound but the intended vowel. Vowels are the part of speech that carry the voice **towards** the listener. This outward movement (opening up for the vowels) is stressed again and again. We combine relaxed jaw, minimal breath, clear voice, lively intonation and outward movement in easy stuttering. Once this is well trained it is a pattern one can and will fall back on in outside situations when spontaneous fluency is threatened, or to help oneself in preventing a stuttering block. It helps to intimately know what is happening, to be able to feel such a block coming, so that one can intervene early in the sequence that leads up to it.

The interval between this stage and the next is at least 6 weeks. Clients are asked to determine their own assignments and make a contract with the group and with themselves. They each choose one other group member to report to regularly. During the interval each client is asked to write to, or telephone the therapist with whom he has had personal consultations at least once as a practical measure to ensure the continuance of therapeutic contacts. In their contracts they are strongly recommended only to name items they are absolutely sure they can accomplish and to name no more than three. They tend to be rather euphoric at this stage and nothing is so conducive to disaster as high demands and expectations. As large promises are the best excuse for no action, we ask for realistic contracts. In this connection we also recommend spending 3 to 5 minutes in concentrated effort several times a day rather than combining the daily training into one much longer session. Keeping a record and reporting developments at the next therapy session are also required.

Clients are encouraged to invite people from their daily environment to participate for varying periods of time during each therapy session: in this way we have "strangers" with us almost every day. The more the outside world comes into the therapy sessions, the more natural it will feel to transfer that which is trained during that time.

Nevertheless there is a distinct disadvantage in intramural group therapy compared to therapy where clients go back to their everyday world after working hours. The intramural group quickly grows to be a safe and warm environment with which the client's ordinary world may then seem to contrast in an unpleasantly cold way. On the other hand, the total acceptance and safety may be just what the stutterer needs to turn the scales so that he can progress towards accepting himself and accepting his stuttering behavior as something for which he is personally responsible.

Stage Four

In the fourth stage the central theme is social interaction. Part of each day is devoted to role playing sessions in which nonverbal action is analyzed. First this is done in standard situations such as asking a favor, refusing a request, contradicting a statement, and so forth. Later we work on situations that express personal difficulties either in the client's job or private life. We stress the value of communication as such — making oneself clear and being willing to listen. Clients first play the situation the way they used to, concentrating on **not** stuttering. The group analyzes and comments on what they see and hear and someone else replays the part so that the protagonist can judge for himself what he wants to change. After every trial the partner(s) in the play are asked for their impressions. Did they feel pushed into the role of a tyrant by the protagonist's obsequious behavior? or threatened by his aggressiveness? Did he seem cold and distant? anxious or vulnerable? It turns out that as the protagonist's behavior changes his partner's does too, quite naturally. In this way clients learn that their own behavior, at least partly, determines the reactions of others. Partners in a conversation are not interested in perfect speech; they want easy communication. As long as the rhythm of normal speech is not disturbed, the listener will quickly adapt to whatever technique the stutterer uses.

In this fourth stage we work on easy stuttering, making the clients change at a given signal from voluntary hard stuttering to easy stuttering and vice versa. Fluency techniques are introduced but only for those who are no longer afraid to stutter openly. We do not stress slow speech very much as this tends to become monotonous and artificial but we do stress the value of pauses. First these pauses come after every three or four words that form a logical unit of thought. We teach the client to exhale very slightly but perceptibly after each such unit but to let inhalation take care of itself. There will always be enough for what one has in mind to say. Gradually these short units are combined to make ordinary sentences. We want the client to be "present" and these pauses give him the opportunity to feel the relaxed alertness of being "all there." The more self-assured and balanced a person becomes, the less he will need to compulsively **inhale** after every couple of words which is such a common phenomenon in many stuttering patterns.

We again ask the client to make a contract. The whole group advises him as to whether they think his contract is realistic or not. As before, the clients work with each other, and report to the therapist. Their reports include what has happened in the situations that have been rehearsed in role playing. Usually these situations will have improved unless they involve deeply emotional relationships in which case more time and work will be needed.

Stage Five

The last stage is a summary of all that has gone before. Part of each day is devoted to bodywork but the training of speech as such becomes more predominant. In this as in former sessions we encourage clients to use their midday break to venture out and "practice" on strangers. We also spend regular therapy time on specific assignments for individual stutterers outside the clinic.

At the end of this basic therapy we advise clients about "refresher courses." Usually two to four out of every group will be able to make it on their own in the future. About half will need one or two extra sessions of five days at six month intervals. Another two or three will need much more, some even as long as five years.

Stuttering is what the stutterer does so as not to stutter, as Sheehan has put it. This is a beautifully concise definition that points in several directions. Stuttering starts as coping behavior under stress: it is an S.O.S. signal from the child to his environment, and then an emergency measure. If the environment understands what is needed to restore balance, all will be well. Otherwise the emergency measures may have to be used so often that they solidify into a habitual defense system. Once this happens the individual grows apprehensive about the reactions to the defense system itself.

Because this defense system comes into being while the individual functions more on the biological level than the social level, I have grown more and more convinced we must return to those levels right at the beginning of therapy. What we do to ensure transfer and maintenance of learned speech behavior depends not on what we do at the end but rather on what we have done **at the beginning** in terms of bodywork. Body concept and self concept have to do with existential and vital energy which can either be blocked in self defense or used constructively in self development. When the stutterer has become aware of his physical self, has become "grounded," he has an added dimension which not only promotes the immediate gain of therapeutic change but increases the likelihood of transfer and maintenance.

Our work on the body concept and self concept level works for everyone, not exclusively stutterers. But stutterers are first of all human beings, so it seems natural to work on what they have in common with all mankind before turning to their specific problem. By organizing therapy in this way we hope to give fluency a better chance to survive in the real world of human communication. A balanced person is a person most likely to make realistic choices and stick to them.

References

Damsté, P. H., "Speech Therapy and Rehabilitation" Volume I in *Disorders of Human Communication*. New York: Springer Verlag Wien, 1983.

Sheehan, Joseph G., "Problems in the Evaluation of Progress and Outcome" in *Seminars in Speech, Language and Hearing*, Volume 1, No. 4, 1980.

Sheehan, Joseph G., "Principles of Therapy" in Gruss, J. Fraser (Ed.), *Counseling Stutterers*. Memphis: Stuttering Foundation of America, 1982.

chapter six

Relapse and Recovery from Stuttering

by Joseph G. Sheehan, Ph.D.

To grow up as a stutterer means, among other things, to experience intervals of relative fluency filled with hope, followed by episodes of blocking filled with despair. We ride the roller coaster of cyclic variation with eternal optimism. In that sense, relapse from fluency is something we have known all our lives. Surely we must have learned something about what makes these intervals seem to come and go, as though we were children of an inexorable fate.

Let's understand that stuttering behavior is lawful behavior. To the layman, what the stutterer does looks like random or disorganized behavior — a hodge-podge. But what the stutterer does is highly patterned, depending to some extent upon the sound characteristics of the word. Stuttering behavior does follow general laws of behavior, even though that fact may not be readily apparent when we are confronted with the sheer irrelevance of the stuttering pattern to the speaking of the word.

Although stutterers exhibit great diversity and are far from being a homogeneous group, most of what we see and observe as stuttering behavior has been learned. The person wasn't born with it. It has a reinforcement history. It didn't just happen.

The stuttering pattern itself is the product of long years of shaping, of the irregular reinforcement of some tricks or grimaces or responses at the expense of others. Learning and conditioning principles underlie both the development of the stuttering pattern, and its perpetuation. The average stutterer is caught in a self-reinforcement pattern, or vicious circle, in which the laws work against him, or against her. Can we learn to identify sources and causes of relapse and to make those laws work for the stutterer, rather than against the stutterer? We believe we can.

Aspects of Relapse

First, we need to consider some dimensions of the problem of stuttering, as experienced by individuals who have that problem. Second, we need to consider varieties and sources of relapse. Third, we need to consider some more or less immediate ways out of relapse and how induction of relapse can lead to ways out of relapse. Fourth, we need to deal with the pervasive and often unrecognized problem of adjusting to improvement or recovery, of accommodating to the unaccustomed role of mostly normal speaker. Frequently that accommodation is more difficult than the adjustment involved in making progress initially.

Dimensions of Stuttering

The handicap of stuttering is fairly divisible into twin aspects of feelings, on one hand, and behavior, on the other. Much of the behavior is visible above the surface and is directly observable to the listener. This is the above-the-surface portion of the iceberg of stuttering — at least, a major part of it.

The feeling portion of the handicap is less accessible to the listener, and may consist of heavy loads of fear, guilt, dejection, and the like. Such feelings do have their behavioral representations, more so in some stutterers than in others.

Public and Private Stuttering

Stuttering is a problem in which efforts at concealment and avoidance become conspicuous aspects of the problem itself. Defensive maneuvers tend to be the most revealing features in any personality; most of us are not well-equipped to conceal our central facets.

Nonetheless, a few stutterers achieve a fine expertise in poker face, poker voice, and poker body language. Such successful denials of the stutterer role become locked into the person's life style, and furnish nutrients for a lush undergrowth of falsity.

Thus stuttering has a public aspect and a private aspect. When we speak of handicap, we must take both into account. Ditto for therapeutic improvement. Ditto for relapse from that improvement. It is astonishing that these two aspects have been so confusingly intermingled in the vast existing literature.

Classical vs. Instrumental Conditioning

The public and private aspects of stuttering, roughly divisible into behavior and feelings, seem to have been acquired on the basis of two different kinds of learning: classical conditioning and instrumental conditioning. Operant conditioning is a term sometimes used for the instrumental type.

The classical or Pavlovian kind of conditioning covers fear or anxiety, guilt and shame, and physiologically involves the sympathetic nervous system with its smooth muscles and gut or viscera. Attitudes and feelings are mostly acquired through this kind of conditioning, and most of that portion of the iceberg under the surface is covered.

Instrumental conditioning covers the motoric or skill side of stuttering, the more or less overt behavior the listener sees. Timing movements, "uhs," facial grimaces, overly wide mouth openings, head movements, forcing or general muscle tension relate more to the instrumental type. But you can't understand stuttering just by looking at those two types of conditioning.

For one thing, the instrumental behaviors are always more available and more easily countable. The feelings of the stutterer are much harder to assess. So in a great many therapy programs, only the outward stuff counts. But we suggest that it's the stutterer who counts, and what's going on inside him that counts even more. That's true for anybody, with or without a handicap: what goes on inside is of central importance.

Suppressive Control

Therapies that aim merely at suppressing the outward occurrence of stuttering tend to do things to the inner occurrence of stuttering. For example, stutterers commonly report that they are sometimes able to "rise to the occasion." They may continue to experience great anxiety about possible stuttering in the situation, but they seem able to suppress or "control" the outward appearance of stuttering behavior.

Even in the absence of suppressive therapies, we find implicit or interiorized stutterers, who have learned suppressive skills extremely well. They don't sound too bad, but they go through agonies of anticipating what might happen. Response suppression has a cost, and the internal cues that mediate stuttering behavior do not automatically vanish because a few moments of stuttering are suppressed.

The kind of person who has the stuttering may be more important than the amount of stuttering the person has. And for a great many people, stuttering is not their worst problem. Too often, clinicians are trained to think of a person who stutters in terms of the frequency of the stuttering behavior. The result is that the person and his or her individuality tends to get lost in the shuffle. In this illusion the clinician is aided and abetted by the stutterer, who frequently suffers from the same misconception.

Attribution

Because stuttering has a sometimes high, if intermittent social visibility, all problems tend to be attributed to it. As part of this attributional set, the feeling aspect of stuttering easily gets ignored. Some experimenters say, we're going to be very scientific and just stick to observables, which is all right to a point. But it's like saying, "We're only going to search for gold where it's convenient for us to search." The inner experiences and feelings of a stutterer are far less accessible to observation, especially in terms of the assessment of results. A notable exception to this unfortunate trend is Gregory's carefully designed assessment of the results of stuttering therapy (Gregory, 1972).

In a broad sense, there is always a psychotherapeutic aspect of therapy for any stutterer, because the person and not just his designated problem should always be the central focus of therapy. The speech-language clinician may still be the therapist of choice, provided that he or she is willing to understand the person. Equally if not more important is a knowledge of the problem of stuttering. This implies interest in more than the block-count.

Avoidance

Stuttering is perpetuated largely by **successful** avoidance. To be sure, not all evasion that is attempted is successful. We fail even at being cowardly. The situation descends upon us, and somehow we flounder through it. Reality forces us to face the task of speaking, even when we're doing it miserably. As a stutterer, you can retreat from speaking and you can forgive yourself for your weakness and cowardice. But the behavioral laws governing stuttering will not be equally forgiving. It's like the unforgiving sea. Make a mistake, and the consequences are relentless. Continue to make them — continue avoiding words and situations — and you have the problem forever. You may let yourself off the hook for the moment, but you build yourself a much bigger problem later on.

You find any stutterer who is still stuttering severely, or who has relapsed, and you'll find that he cheated on the principle of avoidance-reduction. In response to fear or anticipation he weakened and yielded to the temptation to pretend that the problem didn't exist. We are always telling our stutterer's groups, "In a real sense, you continue to stutter because you give up when the going gets tough."

Adaptive Avoidance

Of course, there is an adaptive function to avoidance. We avoid common dangers and it helps us survive. The social situation avoidances of a stutterer can keep him from making a bad impression on his boss, or from being turned down for a date, or from having to deal with the telephone, etc. But avoidance of feared social situations is quite different from avoidance of common dangers, and has different effects. Avoidance of speaking situations tends to increase the fear of the situations avoided, and others like them. When we shrink from the things we fear, we cannot test the reality of what would happen if we gave ourselves a chance to succeed — or to fail. Even when we experience momentary difficulty in tackling fears, there is a meeting of current reality, and an opportunity to profit from that meeting.

Short Steps and Long Goals

It's probably all right for a speaker to avoid a speaking situation, provided he's not a stutterer. If he's a stutterer, then he ought to tackle it, if possible. Of course there are limits to human endurance and courage, and one can carry this Spartan regimen only so far. Neither Rome nor Avoidance-Reduction Therapy was built in a day. Many severe stutterers cannot be expected to head squarely into every challenge that comes along, at least not in the beginning. There is a difference between the ultimate goal, and the smaller steps that lead to it. Challenge/Support ratios and Success/Failure ratios must always be maintained on the side of predominant success. Avoidances usually need to be reduced gradually, and fluency will spread gradually in response. For both the stutterer and the clinician, often it is not courage that is lacking, but patience.

Sources of Relapse

1. False Fluency. This form of fluent experience is so common to stutterers that very few of them ever have to have the term defined. Stutterers themselves tend to be excited only momentarily by episodes or intervals of false fluency, for they know that nothing fundamental has happened. We would define as false, any fluency that results from the successful use of avoidance devices, such as an assumed foreign accent, or clowning behavior. Listeners and sometimes stutterers themselves occasionally delude themselves that such false roles constitute improvement. Relapse in such cases is so certain that the term is hardly applicable. When there has been no real improvement, based on some basic alteration of the stuttering or speaking pattern, or of the cues eliciting these patterns, then return to previous state is automatic. We mention false fluency for the sake of completeness, to portray an illusion probably more common in listeners than in stutterers.

2. Suppressively Based Fluency. Although overlapping with the False Fluency category to some extent, some different processes may be involved. Some stutterers may be observed to exhibit an ability to suppress the outward occurrence of blocking for at least brief periods of time. Since it is not always obvious that distractions are being used, this perhaps deserves separate mention. But response suppression can carry the stutterer only so far. When the level of stimulus complexity builds up beyond threshold, the stutterer experiences "The Return of the Repressed." A reversion to baseline frequency, or usual rate of stuttering, is so inevitable that relapse must be viewed as an integral part of the process.

3. Return of Older Attitudes and Habits (Jost's Law). The basic statement of Jost's Law is that when two habits are of approximately equal strength, but are unequal in age, at any given time in the future the older will be stronger, provided that neither is practiced in the meantime. The newer attitudes and learned behaviors acquired during any kind of therapy tend to be much younger than the handicapping learned behaviors that they have at the moment eclipsed. All the stutterer has to do to relapse is to rest on his oars. The fact that the newer habit is dropping at a much faster rate will ensure that he will have a relapse. That is why some overlearning is typically necessary with any kind of speech therapy, or any kind of psychotherapy as well. Usually, a period of return to the therapy setting for renewal and support is required to strengthen newer and more fragile patterns. The process is similar to what Van Riper calls "stabilization" (Van Riper, 1982).

4. The Strangeness of New Fluency. New roles typically require some adjustment before they replace previously existing patterns of action. As in the case of those with voice problems, new patterns of speaking are not accepted automatically or with ease. First comes a feeling of strangeness and alienation. That which is familiar will feel "right" even though it is objectively wrong, whereas the unfamiliar will feel "wrong" even though it is objectively correct. Such a period of familiarization invites relapse for some time after the acquisition of any new response pattern. We take awhile to get used to ourselves, especially to the sound of improved speaking. In this situation, relapse may masquerade as a return to naturalness.

5. Role Change and Adjustment to Improvement. Even after assimilation of the new sound into the self-concept, there are further adjustments to improvement. Improvement in speaking brings about a new set of expectations. A correction has to be made for the overattribution of all problems to the stuttering handicap. Recovery of fluency may bring about reactions of disappointment. Other problems must be faced, perhaps for the first time.

The assumption that stutterers will easily grasp and hold fluency if it is given to them often turns out to be incredibly naive. Yet that assumption, unrecognized, pervades the maintenance and outcome claims in current literature. That's why often the claims don't hold up when subjected to independent examination or followup.

It is misleading to treat stuttering simply as a problem in behavioral frequency, rather than primarily as the problem of a person. Moreover, stuttering is the problem of a person trying to communicate with other persons. If he has always viewed himself as a "giant in chains," he may not readily accept the realization that he is after all an ordinary mortal with ordinary weaknesses. In psychodynamic terms, this would be described as the loss of the secondary gain component of the stuttering handicap. Despite the heavy primary loss of the ability to communicate, stuttering can be so woven into the life style of the stutterer that change brings new problems.

6. Return to Successful Avoidance. The reinforcement situation is such that the stutterer is immediately rewarded for doing the wrong thing, namely pretending or avoiding, while he is immediately punished or nonreinforced for doing the right thing, namely speaking up and taking part in life. The sheer success of avoidance maneuvers probably is the central perpetuating factor in the problem, and overwhelmingly accounts for the commonness of relapse in the treatment of the disorder.

7. Tragedy, Illness, and Life Stress Events. Possibly as a reminder that life is a constantly changing stream of events, we must note that recovery is never a permanent condition. Human beings can always change, and the world around them can change, and the assumption of constancy never holds.

The medical model term of "cure" implied a permanent respite from a particular illness, often with an immunity against future infections, as with chicken pox or German measles. No such immunity attaches to the future of any speaker who has ever been a stutterer. In fact, even normal speakers may break down under extreme stress conditions such as military combat or catastrophic bereavement.

For improving or recovering stutterers, a certain amount of morale seems required to maintain forward motion, to serve as a countering force to the avoidance tendencies that have been bred into a lifetime of stuttering behavior. When physical illness, the loss of a loved one, or a major disappointment strikes, it would be improbable that some regression in morale and speaking behavior would not occur. Though there is little the clinician can do to prevent tragedies, we must expect that they will take their toll on fluent word production.

A clinical success can always become a failure, just as a clinical failure can always become a success. No human being is ever permanently either.

Relapse Induction and Recovery

The process of therapy is never aimed to be interminable, nor should the stutterer have to be forever dependent upon the clinician for inspiration, ideas and support. Early in therapy, there is a natural dependent relationship between the stutterer and the clinician. For one thing, the stutterer typically arrives full of ignorance and misinformation; the therapist's initial tasks include some direct teaching functions. Otherwise we let the stutterer flounder in the sea of misconception that the public tends to impart.

During therapy the responsibility should shift gradually to the client. He must begin to inform himself and to take action appropriate to the therapy principles or program. Ultimately, if he is to become a success, the stutterer must become his own resource, his own clinician.

Many stutterers who have improved dread the thought of

slipping back, for relapse to any degree seems catastrophic to them. This attitude in itself is a problem in the maintenance of improvement. You can't go through life waiting for the other shoe to drop. It is better for the stutterer to experience some regression or relapse, to analyze the factors or inactions producing it, and to learn how to pull out of it.

Occasionally, we have found it clinically advisable to induce relapse, either through direct suggestion or through "therapy reversal." For example, a stutterer might deliberately go back to avoiding a certain person or a particular speaking situation. The most likely effect is a dramatic increase in fear in the avoided situations, and in other similar situations. He may also experience a general increase in fear and struggle behaviors. After such an experience, going back to the therapy principles may be experienced as a relief, rather than a series of onerous tasks.

One way to get over a fear is to experience what you fear and to discover that the consequences are not irreversible. The "second time around" tends to involve a much greater share of responsibility on the part of the client. He can feel a greater pride in his accomplishment of pulling out of relapse. He has just taken an important step along the road to becoming his own clinician.

The stutterer learns that an occasional fear of a situation or a word does not mean the end of the world, and that an increase in the frequency of blocking need not be treated as a failure. It is better for the stutterer to learn that he need not be perfectly fluent at all times, that speech within an acceptable range is enough, and that some bobbles are best tolerated. That's what normal speakers do!

What the stutterer needs is not speech that is stumble-free or stutter-free, but speech that is avoidance-free. Yet that can come naturally, and should require no special effort. Without avoidance of words or situations, the stutterer can be himself. And he can be himself with ever widening circles of fluency — not perfect — just normal or acceptable. No therapy can be judged a success or complete if the person must maintain an eternal vigilance over the mechanics of speech production. The ultimate aim of therapy should be to produce an independence of the therapist, just as the eventual aim of every parent should be to produce a child that can become his own person.

References

Boberg, Einer, "Maintenance of Fluency: An Experimental Program" in Boberg, E. (Ed.), *Maintenance of Fluency: Proceedings of the Banff Conference*, New York: Elsevier North-Holland, 1981.

Conture, Edward, *Stuttering*. Englewood Cliffs, NJ: Prentice-Hall, 1982.

Erickson, Robert L., "Assessing Communication Attitudes Among Stutterers" in *Journal of Speech and Hearing Research*, 12, 711-723, 1969.

Fraser, Malcolm, *Self-Therapy for the Stutterer* (revised). Memphis: Stuttering Foundation of America, 1983.

Gregory, Hugo H. (Ed.), *Controversies About Stuttering Therapy*. Baltimore: University Park Press, 1979.

Gruss, Jane Fraser (Ed.), *Counseling Stutterers*. Memphis: Stuttering Foundation of America, 1982.

Perkins, William H. (Ed.), *Strategies in Stuttering Therapy*. Stuttgart and New York: Thieme-Stratton, 1980.

Sheehan, Joseph G., "Principles of Therapy" in Gruss, J. F. (Ed.), *Counseling Stutterers*. Memphis: Stuttering Foundation of America, 1982.

Van Riper, C. G., *The Nature of Stuttering* (revised). Englewood Cliffs, NJ: Prentice-Hall, 1982.

Versteegh-Vermeij, Elisabeth, "Body Concept, Self Concept and Balance" in Gruss, J. F. (Ed.), *Stuttering Therapy: Transfer and Maintenance*. Memphis: Stuttering Foundation of America, 1983.

Williams, Dean E., "Stuttering" in Curtis, James F. (Ed.), *Human Communication: Basic Processes and Disorders*. New York: Harper & Row, 1978.

chapter seven

Commentary

by Hugo H. Gregory, Ph.D.

In this final chapter, I will attempt to highlight topics discussed at the conference and emphasized by the authors of the preceding chapters. Some of my own ideas and experiences will be shared.

Attitude Change

We agree that attitudinal (cognitive-affective) changes influence in an important way the transfer and maintenance of more overt speech improvement. In fact, discussion at the conference focused almost equally on issues and procedures related to speech modification and attitude change. In this connection, Boberg (1981) noted that speakers at another conference on the maintenance of fluency, speakers who had been associated mainly with overt speech change during the decade of the 1970s, referred frequently to the consideration of attitudes associated with effective maintenance.

Conture[1] gives clinicians an understanding of some of the

---

[1]In this chapter where no reference is given, the reference is to the author's chapter in this book.

patterns of thinking in stutterers that contribute to the success or failure of therapy. He describes "Joe" who felt rejected by listeners, a perception that was a projection of his own self-rejecting attitude. Conture believes this attitude was a major factor in Joe's failure to transfer improved fluency. Sheehan reminds us of the sensitivity that stutterers have about disfluency, something we can readily understand. The desire to conceal and avoid quickly becomes a major part of the problem. Furthermore, stutterers may attribute all their problems to stuttering. Boberg, Conture, Sheehan, and Versteegh offer examples of attitudinal factors that need attention. Versteegh emphasizes getting to know the individual characteristics of a stutterer, getting beyond the overt speech behaviors to the "boiler room." Her experience convinces her that a stutterer's learning to acknowledge and express feelings more openly is an essential element in effective stuttering therapy. Stutterers in therapy are not just changing speakers, they are people who are adjusting to new opportunities and responsibilities.

With specific reference to transfer and maintenance, I believe it is important for stutterers to realize clearly the process nature of change. When adult stutterers have been stuttering for years, they ordinarily understand that a three-week or a three-month program of therapy is not going to be all that is required. When we describe therapy to clients, we should explain the need for maintenance activities, as I say to clients, for 12-18 months following the course of therapy, and to a lesser extent thereafter. One reason, not the only one of course, that we see some stutterers for therapy who have already been to several clinics, is that they hoped for and were perhaps led to believe that treatment was shorter term than it usually is. Speech and attitudinal changes require time for integration into an individual's personality. I now say to stutterers, "Let this be your last therapy. This means participating in follow-up activities for 12-18 months after the period of formal therapy." Returning to the clinic for review sessions must be viewed as a positive thing to do, not a sign of weakness.

Boberg recommends the following attitude for a client to have while focusing on maintenance: *Clients should approach friends and family with the attitude that they are very pleased with the progress they have achieved on their speech but that there is still some way to go."*

Accepting New Behavior

Over the years, I have talked with stutterers and individuals with other speech and voice problems about the difficulty of accepting change. I may say, "You came here to change, to stutter less, but now that you can modify your speech and speak with more normal fluency, it seems strange. It's not you. You are more used to the old you who stuttered." Then, I explain that we as clinicians can understand this. We all need time to adjust to modified behavior.

Williams tells us that children feel conspicuous when they act in ways in which they are not used to acting. He emphasizes the importance of people in the environment knowing what changes the child is making so they can be supportive. Positive reinforcement for "new behavior" helps greatly in generating a positive attitude.

Sheehan warns that relapse may masquerade as a return to naturalness. He points out, "That which is familiar will feel 'right' even though it is objectively wrong, whereas the unfamiliar will feel 'wrong' even though it is objectively correct."

Listening to an audiotape recording of their speech has always been valuable in helping stutterers adjust to change. Watching and listening to audio-video recordings appears to be even more effective. Children and adult clients have reported that they gradually begin to like their new behavior.

Finally, I believe that viewing change as a continuing activity helps in accepting and enjoying change. In my opinion, it is better not to speak of "speech modifications." This may lead stutterers to believe that they will learn certain modifications and then the job will be done. It is better to refer to "modifying speech," a process subjects can find interesting and rewarding for the rest of their lives. For example, at a certain point, the more specific objective may be to link words smoothly in phrases. Later, modifying speech may focus on better inflection, variation in rate, and so forth.

Experiencing Regression

This topic was discussed at length and the conference participants agreed that it is important for stutterers to realize that degrees of relapse will occur and that one can recover. A great deal can be learned from this experience. First, stutterers can gain additional insight into the cyclic nature of stuttering. While steady improvement can be expected, there will be some ups and downs. They should not panic when some regression occurs. Experiencing recovery reduces the fear associated with degrees of relapse that are certain to occur. Secondly, this gives stutterers the opportunity to problem solve, to determine what factors may have resulted in this temporary set-back. If the basis for therapy is a "stutter more fluently" approach, did they begin to slip back into the old habit of avoiding words and situations, of being overly sensitive about disfluency? If the basis for therapy is a "speak more fluently" approach, did they not keep the fluency-producing skills vividly in mind through regular practice? If the basis for therapy is a combination of these two approaches, stutterers can think about how well non-avoidance procedures and normal speech fluency skills have been utilized. In connection with this, when a stutterer increases fluency there may be a tendency for the desire to avoid disfluency and stuttering to increase. This is true whether the approach is a "speak more fluently" or a "stutter more fluently" one (Gregory 1979). I believe it is crucial for stutterers to have insight into this tendency. In combining the two approaches, stutterers can increase fluency skills (approach behavior) and at the same time minimize avoidance feelings by knowing how to modify stuttering as it occurs, and perhaps by using some voluntary disfluency.

Perkins warns that what he calls lucky fluency can lead to degrees of relapse. All of us who have worked with stutterers or have stuttered ourselves can understand why stutterers love fluency that comes without effort. We also know that this fluency is usually short term. This lucky fluency, or "flight into fluency," as I have termed it, that often occurs during therapy, probably results from the surge of relief from fear and feeling of increased confidence that comes from experiencing more fluency and having increased hope of overcoming stuttering. We know that when life circumstances are particularly good for a stutterer not in therapy, they may also experience periods of greatly increased fluency. The cyclic nature of stuttering is still not understood well, but stutterers need to know that these cycles occur during and after therapy, as well as before!

Perkins prefers to have a stutterer find out while still in therapy that lucky fluency is not lasting and to have that person learn speaking skills that enhance the production and maintenance of fluency. Likewise, Sheehan believes it essential for a stutterer to learn that what he terms "false fluency" is not based on any basic alteration of the stuttering or speaking pattern, or the cues associated with these patterns.

Planning Transfer

There is general agreement that as therapy progresses specific attention should be given to the planning of activities aimed toward enabling a school aged child or an adult to change behavior in progressively more natural environmental situations. Among the conference participants, Boberg and Williams were the most specific in describing these procedures. As they talked about what they do, the others frequently said, "I do that too."

In discussing children, Williams states, "The essence of therapy is to help the child cope constructively with his speech production abilities in the presence of emotional feelings involved in his everchanging communicative interactions." He emphasizes the communication nature of a stuttering problem. Thus, the clinician in the school has to relate to the child's teacher in light of the child's activities in the classroom. Williams offers practical advice about working effectively with teachers and parents. For example, the clinician can discuss with the teacher ways she would feel comfortable participating in the therapy program. Transfer for the child is not going to be effective if the clinician relates ineffectively with the teacher, and all teachers are different!

The clinician's objective is for the teacher to understand what the child is working on and to be supportive. Interestingly, Williams warns that the teacher should not be expected to correct or modify the child's speech. Speaking of the teacher he says, "She can provide the opportunities for the child to speak and she can observe his performance. She should not be expected to directly correct or modify the child's speech . . . one clinician is enough."

We all agreed with Williams that children are more successful in therapy if they know that teachers and parents, and perhaps some peers understand what they are doing. I will discuss my own experience with this in a section to follow on working with pre-school children. There is agreement with Williams' description of transfer procedures relating to language — propositionality complexity, social complexity, and reaction complexity.

Boberg recognizes the desirability of certain personalized transfer activities as well as ones that are generally standard from person to person. Standard transfers are described in a presumed hierarchy of difficulty. Boberg notes that some clients need more careful guidance in carrying out transfer assignments and some require more practice in the clinic before they are ready for transfer situations.

For many years we have recognized that one of the clinicians' major responsibilities is to arrange gradations of experiences that are conducive to effective learning (Gregory 1968, Van Riper 1973). Boberg has helped us to be more specific about transfer procedures in the treatment of stuttering.

Self-monitoring and Evaluation

The effectiveness of therapy in improving a stutterer's self-monitoring skills is seen as important in determining how successful a client is in transfer and maintenance. Some therapy programs adopt the position that unadaptive stuttering behavior needs to be monitored and changed in such a way that stutterers become better acquainted with the topography of their stuttering. Other therapy programs emphasize the monitoring of speech gestures that result in increased fluency. Early in therapy clinicians and clients work together as clients learn to monitor what they do as they stutter or as they modify their speech. Clinicians may model this monitoring for the clients. For example, clinicians may feign stuttering blocks with varying amounts of tension and repeat these blocks showing stutterers how to monitor and imitate the behavior. As therapy progresses, clinicians encourage clients to be more independent in self-assessment. As an illustration, if clients are identifying occurrences of stuttering in their speech, clinicians may first signal instances of stuttering in the clients' speech, followed by both clinicians and clients noting occurrences of stuttering and the amount of agreement between judgments, and finally the clients making independent judgments. In this way, the monitoring of stuttering is learned.

When the target behavior is a way of modifying stuttering or modifying speech, the clinician may at first reinforce the stutterer's modified behavior, then both the client and clinician signal the correct behavior and note agreement, followed by the stutterer's reinforcing his own correct modification. If these monitoring and self-evaluation procedures are taught precisely during the modification stages of therapy, they can be more readily extended during transfer and after formal therapy ends.

Conture emphasizes the advantages (to transfer) of giving a stutterer immediate feedback about speech production using electromyography and electroglottography. The more effective stutterers are in monitoring their behavior, the more likely it is that they will be able to monitor sufficiently when under emotional stress.

Finally, Boberg tells us how stutterers in his program are responsible for analyzing their own transfer tapes with reference to which words are stuttered, which ones are cancelled correctly, correct phrasing, rate, easy onsets, etc.

Intensiveness of Therapy

We concluded in our discussions that therapy had to be fairly intensive during the beginning stages and gradually tapered off to less intensive and finally infrequent, depending on the individual. Williams says that a child receiving therapy in a school situation should be seen for a minimum of two or three sessions, 30-40 minutes in length, per week. If more frequent sessions are needed to meet the child's needs, they should be scheduled. Williams stresses that if this cannot be done, the child should be referred to someone who can meet the child's needs.

In terms of what we know about stuttering as a behavior involving fear associated behaviors, we cannot hope to accomplish sufficient counter-conditioning unless therapy is frequent enough for the child or adult to realize some change in a short period of time. In work with adults, I have found that a minimum of three one-hour sessions a week is necessary at the beginning of therapy. In our combined group and individual therapy program, adult stutterers are in therapy two hours a day for each of two or three days a week. Some other programs are very intensive, that is, four to six hours a day for several weeks. Versteegh described a program in which therapy consists of 5 sessions of 5 days each, spaced with increased intervals to cover six months. After this, follow-up sessions of 5 days are offered, depending on the person's needs.

We discussed how the clinician makes the decision to move to less intensive treatment sessions. This is a decision that has to take into consideration the individual nature of the client's problem and progress made. I have found that moving to less frequent sessions can be a reward to the client for progress made. I say, "Keep this up and you can cut down to one session a week." I hasten to add that the clinician must continue to see the client at least once a week during the crucial period of increased transfer, not only to check on speech change, but also, in my experience, to help clients profit from attitude-oriented therapy as they experience more comfortable communication and increased freedom from stuttering. This is in agreement with Sheehan's and Versteegh's emphasis that behavioral, cognitive, and affective changes have to be integrated during and following therapy.

Planning Maintenance

One of my first professors said to me, "You know I think we tend to dismiss stutterers from therapy when we see that they can cope with their stuttering. In fact, this is probably the time when they can begin to make the most progress of all. Stutterers need to stay involved in therapy for a rather long period of time." I have thought many times about this statement made in 1951 by Harold Westlake.

More and more in recent years, the need for specific activities aimed toward helping stutterers extend therapeutic change has been recognized and provided. Boberg has described a maintenance program consisting of a variety of scheduled clinic visits and a home program. Clinic visits take a variety of forms including evening visits, refresher weekends, and five day booster sessions. The home program includes speech assignments, self-evaluations, and daily speech recordings. This program sounds rather demanding! However, follow-up of clients has shown that stutterers find it difficult to stay motivated and continue therapy on their own unless they have these specifically planned home programs and scheduled recheck sessions. This is certainly understandable to all of us who have undertaken personal improvement programs such as regular physical exercise or weight-loss. We concluded that a stutterer should not enter a therapy program that does not include transfer activities and a planned maintenance regimen.

References

Boberg, I. (Ed.), *Maintenance of Fluency*. New York: Elsevier, 1981.

Gregory, H., "Applications of Learning Theory Concepts in the Management of Stuttering," in Gregory, H. (Ed.), *Learning Theory and Stuttering Therapy*. Evanston: Northwestern University Press, 1968.

Gregory, H., "Controversial Issues: Statement and Review of the Literature," in Gregory, H. (Ed.), *Controversies About Stuttering Therapy*. Baltimore: University Park Press, 1979.

Gregory, H., "The Controversies: Analysis and Current Status," in Gregory, H. (Ed.), *Controversies About Stuttering Therapy*. Baltimore: University Park Press, 1979.

Sheehan, J., "Problems in the Evaluation of Progress and Outcome," in Perkins, W. (Ed.), *Strategies in Stuttering Therapy*. New York: Thieme-Stratton, 1980.

Van Riper, C., *The Treatment of Stuttering*. Englewood Cliffs, NJ: Prentice Hall, 1973.